THE SENSATIONAL
Toddler
Sleep Plan

www.**penguin**.co.uk

Also by Alison Scott-Wright

The Sensational Baby Sleep Plan

THE SENSATIONAL
Toddler
Sleep Plan

A PRACTICAL GUIDE TO SLEEP-RICH
AND STRESS-FREE PARENTING

ALISON SCOTT-WRIGHT

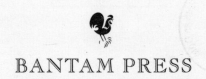

BANTAM PRESS

TRANSWORLD PUBLISHERS
Penguin Random House, One Embassy Gardens,
8 Viaduct Gardens, London SW11 7BW
www.penguin.co.uk

Transworld is part of the Penguin Random House group of companies
whose addresses can be found at global.penguinrandomhouse.com

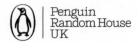

First published in Great Britain in 2021 by Bantam Press
an imprint of Transworld Publishers

The information in this book reflects the author's own opinions and methods, but is not
intended as a substitute for advice from a qualified medical practitioner. Always consult a
qualified medical practitioner before starting, changing or stopping any medical treatment
or making any changes to your child's diet. So far as the author is aware, the information
given is correct and up to date as at date of publication. Practice, laws and regulations all
change, and the reader should obtain up-to-date professional advice on any such issues.
The author and publishers disclaim, as far as the law allows, any liability arising directly
or indirectly from the use, or misuse, of the information contained in this book.

Every effort has been made to obtain the necessary permissions with
reference to copyright material, both illustrative and quoted. We apologize
for any omissions in this respect and will be pleased to make the
appropriate acknowledgements in any future edition.

A CIP catalogue record for this book
is available from the British Library.

ISBN 9781787635067

Typeset in Birka by Palimpsest Book Production Ltd, Falkirk, Stirlingshire.
Printed and bound in Great Britain by Clays Ltd, Elcograf S.p.A.

The authorized representative in the EEA is Penguin Random House Ireland,
Morrison Chambers, 32 Nassau Street, Dublin D02 YH68.

Penguin Random House is committed to a sustainable
future for our business, our readers and our planet. This book
is made from Forest Stewardship Council® certified paper.

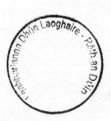

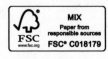

MIX
Paper from
responsible sources
FSC
www.fsc.org   FSC® C018179

This dedication is twofold. Firstly it is to my daughter, Chelsea, who has blossomed into an amazing young woman. She has long been my rock and was especially supportive while I was writing this book, for which I am truly grateful.

Secondly this dedication is to all my wonderful clients and followers, many of whom have become very dear friends. Your continued endorsement – and purchase of multiple copies of *The Sensational Baby Sleep Plan* for your pregnant friends – has directly led to this sequel. I must also mention your many thousand babies and children who have happily responded to my sleep-training and routines, and shown how easily they can sleep well when given the opportunity.

Contents

Foreword by Millie Mackintosh   ix

Introduction   1

Chapter 1: Sleep Matters   7

Chapter 2: Toddler Development and Parenting Tips   25

Chapter 3: Developmental Changes and Sleep   63

Chapter 4: Before You Start Sleep-training   103

Chapter 5: The Reassurance Sleep-training Technique   123

Chapter 6: Siblings, Travel and the Toilet   179

Chapter 7: Reflux and Food Intolerances   213

Sources   253

Acknowledgements   259

Index   261

FOREWORD

by Millie Mackintosh

It is no exaggeration to say that Alison's first book, *The Sensational Baby Sleep Plan*, was an absolute game-changer for me and for my baby daughter. It was a helping hand when we needed it most, a wise voice that rose above the noise, and a guide that offered me some semblance of control when everything felt overwhelming. It is no small thing to find yourself suddenly responsible for a lovely little human, and at times the challenges of those early months felt immense. I turned to Alison's book on a really bad day, and it gave me hope. I have since recommended it to many new parents, and they have come back to me in their droves to say thank you and that it was a game-changer for them too. If you've already read it, then you'll likely know what I'm talking about!

But, much as we'd like to believe otherwise, there are always new bumps in the road of infant sleep. Your napping newborn is suddenly a one-year-old, and they don't need quite as many naps now. Perhaps they aren't sleeping at night as well as they once did. Or they never really found their routine. While Alison's first book was my sleep bible for the first year of my daughter's life, I am so relieved that *The Sensational Toddler Sleep Plan* is now here to see us through the next few years. For all the parents who found help in *The Sensational Baby Sleep Plan*, this is the book that will keep you on track. And for those who haven't read the first book and who have either been struggling with sleep for over a year or who have hit a difficult patch, this is the book that will fix things for you!

There are stories from other parents who have been helped by Alison in these pages – and I hope that by the end of this book you'll have your own story too – but I wanted to share mine here.

We knew before she was born that Sienna was a breech baby (in her case, she was positioned with her head above her feet) and that this is known to sometimes cause hip problems in a child. We were therefore offered a routine scan when she was twelve weeks old to check how her hips were developing. We weren't expecting any issues, so we left that appointment feeling shocked and quite distressed: we'd been told that she had hip dysplasia and were given a harness that she had to wear for 24 hours every day for at least the following six weeks. It was horrible to see our cuddly little girl with her legs strapped up and to the side like a frog. She was very uncomfortable for the first few days, and I felt miserable that I couldn't make it better for her.

I expected things to improve as Sienna got used to being in that position, but that wasn't at all the case. Instead, the things that had been difficult beforehand – the sleepless nights, the crying, the fussy feeding – all became much more challenging. I knew that Sienna had previously displayed some of the symptoms of reflux, but I'd never been particularly worried, and we'd been told time and again that all babies struggle to sleep and that there was nothing unusual about a particularly tricky 'witching hour' in the evenings. But the fixed position of the harness exacerbated every symptom, and in the evenings she now cried for hours before eventually falling asleep, completely exhausted.

I was so grateful when a lovely friend whose child had also experienced hip dysplasia and sleeplessness reached out to offer support. In our conversation, she mentioned a book that had been hugely helpful: *The Sensational Baby Sleep Plan*. I bought it straight away. I was desperate to find a solution and to help my poor daughter. She wasn't sleeping well at all, which meant that she was overtired, and that in turn made her even more miserable! And, if I'm honest, I was struggling too. I'm not ashamed to admit that there were tears from both of us on quite a few occasions. I felt so guilty, like I ought to be doing more to help her. And the lack of sleep was very challenging. I was lost in a fog, doing stupid things (like putting my coffee in the freezer!) and feeling completely detached from myself.

In *The Sensational Baby Sleep Plan* Alison covers so much more than just sleep – much as she does in this new book – so that her readers can be absolutely sure that they are doing the right thing for their child. I remember reading about the signs and symptoms of reflux, and recognizing almost every single one in my daughter. I reached out to Alison, and she called me almost straight away. She promised that things would get better; all the information was in the book and she was on hand to help me too.

The relief was incredible.

With Alison's guidance, we saw a doctor who prescribed medication to assist with reflux, and the change in Sienna was almost instantaneous. She was calm, settled and so much happier. She couldn't have slept while so uncomfortable, and I'm so grateful that we were given the right tools with which to help her. Her sleep gradually began to improve, but we still had no routine whatsoever, which meant that planning our days was very difficult. I was also really keen to have my evenings back; I wanted some time to myself to unwind after such full-on days and to eat dinner with my husband again!

I knew that Sienna wasn't uncomfortable any more, so I felt that it was the right time for us, as a family, to start focusing on a routine. Alison gave us some further advice and encouraged us to use the tools outlined in her book. After a few days, Sienna was sleeping through the night. I cannot tell you how incredible it feels to have your first full night's sleep in months. And it takes so little time to get there!

I started to feel more and more like myself again. It was as though the fog was lifting and, once it had gone, I was happy and relaxed. We had a regular routine for our daytimes, peaceful evenings, and we were all sleeping solidly through the night. And, of course, Sienna was happier than ever too. She clearly had more energy and it was so reassuring to see how smiley she'd become. I look at my daughter now and she isn't a baby any more, but almost a toddler. I am so enjoying watching her lovely little personality emerge, and she's discovering that she has her own wants and that she can push our boundaries with her cheeky smile.

Alison remains a wonderful source of support and guidance for me and my family. We have had bumps in the road and it is inevitable that there will be more going forwards; typically, as soon as we've mastered one stage, something new comes along. I am so relieved that we'll have *The Sensational Toddler Sleep Plan* in hand when she decides that she wants to read just one more book or have just one more sip of water before going to bed!

But our next challenge is likely even closer than that. Sienna will soon be coming off her medication and there's a chance that this will affect her sleep. I don't feel nervous about it this time, though, which is all thanks to Alison. I know that this book has the answers to guide me going forwards and that we have good, solid sleep ahead. With this book by your side, you do too!

I wish you the best of luck, and the soundest of sleep.

Millie Mackintosh, 2021

Introduction

My first book, *The Sensational Baby Sleep Plan*, was published in 2010, and since then many thousands of parents who follow and believe in my methods have asked, 'Where's your next book, Alison?'

And, at last, here it is: *The Sensational Toddler Sleep Plan*.

It is designed not just for those who have used my first book, but for all parents of young children – those with older babies, toddlers and preschoolers who want to ensure they establish and endorse long-term positive sleep associations for their little ones.

I started out specializing in baby sleep but quickly realized that there was little point helping a baby to sleep in a household where older siblings were still waking up throughout the night. And so I expanded my work to cover resolving all childhood sleep problems. I often joked with my clients: 'It's pay for one and get an extra one or two free!'

Over the past few years it's been widely reported that sleep problems in toddlers and children are on the increase. One report claimed that sleep deprivation is a 'hidden health crisis' – and that's based only on recorded cases! This particular study was reported in the *Guardian* using data analysed from NHS Digital, the national information and technology partner to the health and social care system in England.

I know that childhood sleep problems are increasing dramatically, having witnessed first-hand the ever-growing number of parents who are struggling to get their babies, toddlers and young children to sleep. Over the past few generations the new and accepted attitude to infant sleep is simply that babies won't, don't and can't learn to do it, and certainly not before six or even twelve months of age. So a lack of sleep has become the norm and, although we are all aware how detrimental this is to a child's health and development, there never seems to be an answer for how to change things.

My first book addresses the sleep issues that many parents face in those first few months and sets out a plan that, if followed, will result in your baby naturally sleeping 12 hours through the night by around eight to twelve weeks old. The book also details my incredibly popular reassurance sleep-training technique. It was originally aimed at babies aged three to four months and designed for those still sleeping in a cot. However, from twelve months on, as babies develop and head towards toddlerhood, sleeping – even in a cot – can present many different challenges. They've learned to sit up, stand up, use words, throw their comforter, refuse bedtime milk, demand one more story, beg and plead you to sit with them, insist on having the door open and a light on, undo their sleeping bag, take off their pyjamas and – horror – even remove their nappy! Thankfully, the technique and advice detailed in this book will ensure solid sleep for your older babies and toddlers too.

A PARENT'S STORY

'I had no idea what to do when my previously dream-sleeping baby woke one night and started calling for Mama. She was two-and-a-half years old and I couldn't work out what the problem was; there seemed no reason. I went in and tried to soothe her, cuddled her, offered water, but she seemed reluctant to go back into her cot. I hoped it was a one-off, but sadly that wasn't to be. It escalated each night and, after two exhausting and exasperating weeks, I called Alison. After talking things through in detail, Alison felt that my daughter didn't want to be in a cot any more. I was terrified of putting her in a bed, imagining her roaming free around the house. Needless to say, Alison talked me through the whole process and, by the second night of being in the new bed, Harriet was sleeping happily again and has done to this day!'

V. H.

This book will explain how to manage all of the above and more, guiding you through every aspect of sleep for children over one year of age. You will learn about the science of your toddler's sleep, how sleep habits change during natural developmental phases and about other factors that can affect their sleep.

The book addresses many 'sleep problems' and how and why they occur, but most importantly it explains how to resolve them using my renowned reassurance sleep-training technique. This popular method has been successfully used by thousands of parents, who find that reassuring their unsettled child with intermittent visits to the room and comforting words, along with clear boundaries for bedtime, has brought quick and easy resolution – and sound sleep for the whole family. The book explains in detail how to implement reassurance sleep-training with confidence and ease, so you, too, can help your toddler to sleep well and independently. You will also learn to better understand your toddler so you can work out the underlying cause of their sleep problems or why things seem to have gone off-track, and will soon be equipped with the knowledge and tools to find the resolution yourself. The last chapter provides detailed information on acid-reflux, dietary intolerances and food allergies in older babies and children, which are often at the root of children's sleep problems and may be resolved relatively easily.

My method has worked wonders for so many families and in just a few days their little ones are happily going to bed and sleeping right through the night.

In this book you will learn how to manage:

- bedtimes

- sleep patterns

- daytime naps

- night feeds
- night-time waking
- milk feeds
- weaning off milk
- developmental changes
- sleep regressions
- siblings
- removing the dummy
- seasonal hour changes
- travel across time-zones
- illnesses
- teething
- toilet issues
- the transition to a bed
- gastro-oesophageal reflux
- dietary intolerances and allergies

ALISON SAYS . . .

'Many parents have said that they find my calm and confident manner incredibly reassuring and are so grateful to have my advice, as it seems to be the only advice that actually makes sense! They also say that when their toddler has an unexpected night-time wake-up, they'll say to themselves, "What would Alison say or do?", and with my words ringing in their ears, they are easily able to manage the situation. I really do hope that you, too, will find my advice invaluable and be able to emulate and adopt my calm, reassuring approach.'

CHAPTER 1

Sleep Matters

Quite bizarrely, the actual concept of achieving any degree of sleep when you become a parent is often spoken about with derision and almost ridiculed, as it is generally accepted that sleep is likely to be elusive for months, and even years, to come. However, sleep is an essential part of maintaining good all-round health throughout the animal kingdom – and that includes parents and their little ones. During sleep, the body restores the immune, nervous, skeletal and muscular systems, a process that is vital for maintaining mood, memory and cognitive function while awake and also plays a big role in supporting the endocrine (hormone) system. This chapter will explain further why we need to sleep and what happens when we don't, and gives some key tips for promoting wonderful, restorative and necessary sleep for your little one.

SLEEP SCIENCE

As humans living on Planet Earth, we follow a natural day–night split ruled by the sun and the moon. Our sleep–wake cycles are set by light and dark, which influence our naturally-occurring biological rhythms.

ALISON SAYS . . .

'Having been in relative darkness in the womb, babies, once born, take only a few weeks to balance their sleep hormones. By implementing some simple steps you can stimulate them to sleep more at night and have their wakeful periods during the day. By eight to twelve weeks they are capable of sleeping a full 11–12-hour night, but if your toddler has not yet mastered the art, don't panic – it's never too late!'

We produce two sleep hormones that are essential in order for our body to get into a good sleep rhythm. Melatonin, known as 'the sleep trigger', is produced in a higher quantity as we wind down for bed and peaks as we settle to sleep. Cortisol, known as 'the stress hormone', is the opposite: it actually wakes us up.

To go to sleep, we need higher levels of melatonin, but after a few hours of sleep the melatonin levels in our system start to drop as cortisol production begins. Our levels of cortisol continue to rise as the morning approaches and peak around 8am, ensuring that we wake up. There is a natural crossover point during the night as the levels of these important sleep hormones gently ebb and flow, but if cortisol is overproduced we will either find it difficult to fall asleep at bedtime or we will wake in the early hours and struggle to go back to sleep.

In adults, an excess of cortisol is caused mainly by stress, but for babies and children the main cause of too much cortisol is – believe it or not – sleep deprivation. This can be a tricky situation to escape from because, for little ones, sleep deprivation causes stress and, as in adults, this can increase cortisol levels too. It's a vicious circle. Mistakenly, many parents think that if they limit their child's sleep during the day they will sleep better at night, but this actually has the opposite effect as the child will get overtired, and therefore stressed, and thus produce more cortisol!

ALISON SAYS . . .

'For as long as I can remember one of my main mantras has been "Sleep breeds sleep", and it has been proven to me time and time again by all the parents who follow my ethos and wholeheartedly agree!'

When adults get tired, generally they will relax and slow down, but children just get more active and wired. If your toddler is going to bed too late in the evening, is regularly waking early and not napping enough throughout the day, it doesn't necessarily mean that they have had enough sleep: it usually means the opposite. By implementing some simple steps that are explained further in this book, the balance can be reverted. As better sleep becomes established, the sleep-banks fill and the cortisol levels drop to a more normal level quite quickly.

The importance of sleep

A child's brain is utterly amazing and will triple in weight between birth and the age of two! This is why the first two years are the most formative and critical period of a child's development.

No pressure, then! Most parents already feel overwhelmed with so much conflicting advice about how to look after their baby or toddler. However, there's no need to panic, as your little one's requirements are mainly uncomplicated. There are a few simple but key steps to remember, all of which will promote well-being in all areas of emotional, psychological, physical and cognitive development:

- Offer as much calm, positive and peaceful love as possible, with lots of physical contact, cuddles and hugs.

- Engage with them on all levels, through chatting, watching and listening. Pay positive attention rather than offering a distracted interaction.

- Provide a calm and happy home without anger, arguments, shouting or negativity.

- Understand how to give emotional and positive endorsements to your child.

- Limit screen time – *yours* as well as your child's!

- Ensure some fresh air and exercise each day.

- Implement a simple daily routine – your child will feel safe and secure if they know what's coming next each day.

- Create boundaries and limits, and try to be consistent.

- Establish a bath-and-bedtime routine at the end of each day.

- Ensure your child gets enough rest, because sleep is of paramount importance and will keep everything else on track. Without proper rest your little one will struggle to function on a number of levels.

Sleep is an essential building block for a child's mental and physical health, and it plays a crucial role in the development of young minds. In addition to having a direct effect on happiness, research also shows that sleep impacts alertness and attention, cognitive performance, mood, resilience, vocabulary acquisition, learning and memory. Sleep also has an important effect on growth, especially in early infancy. For toddlers, daytime napping is also reported to be necessary for memory consolidation, focus, attention and motor-skill development.

Sleep deprivation

If you're finding it impossible to help your toddler sleep, you're certainly not alone. The American Academy of Pediatrics estimates that sleep problems affect 25–50 per cent of children and 40 per cent of adolescents. Understanding your child's sleep-needs is the first step towards providing better sleep for them. Through a combination of good sleep hygiene, age-appropriate routines, close attention to any sleep disorders or underlying digestive issues, and by following my book, you can help your child get the rest and sleep they need to grow up strong and healthy.

Sleep deprivation in the early months and years takes a toll on all aspects of a child's health and, if not resolved, can have a hugely detrimental effect on their development. Sleep is such an important part of your child's mental and physical health because, while sleeping, a child's mind and body are able to rest and rejuvenate. The brain needs to sleep so that it can restore resources that were used up during the day, and a well-rested brain can solve problems, learn new information and enjoy life much more than a brain that is overtired. The body, too, functions poorly without proper sleep – among other problems, tiredness can impair both hormone production and neurological responses. Thankfully, these are easily reversible with a full night's sleep.

This is easily understood when you read the list below of the signs and symptoms of sleep deprivation for different age ranges:

Younger babies

- A lack of interest in people and the immediate environment

- A tendency to look away from stimulating things

- Repetitive hand-to-face gestures such as ear-pulling and eye-rubbing

- Fluttering eyelids

- Yawning

- Difficulty feeding

- Excessive crying

Older babies and toddlers

- Becoming more 'clingy'

- Protesting at necessary tasks such as nappy changing

- Displaying irritability and moodiness

- Seeming to be very accident-prone

- Being very active in their sleep, often moving around the cot or bed

- Appearing tired throughout the day even though they seem to sleep at night, most likely because they are very active in their sleep

- Trouble with feeding and a disinterest in solid food

- Prone to sudden outbursts of crying for no apparent reason

Older children

- Inability to control emotions

- Having a lack of focus and concentration

- Low motivation and a lack of self-esteem

- Difficulty learning and absorbing new information

- Struggling in social environments

- Headaches and blurred vision

- Extreme mood swings

- Impaired or lower immunity

- Dietary issues, which might lead to 'fussy eating' or obesity

- Anxiety, stress and depression

Meanwhile, babies, toddlers and children who consistently get a good night's sleep tend to display the following behaviours:

Younger babies

- Smile more and engage with facial interaction

- Feed well and enjoy their milk feeds

- Rarely cry

- Are happy and content to be left for short periods

Older babies and toddlers

- Happily entertain themselves

- Are quite chilled, relaxed and rarely 'protest' at anything

- Enjoy fast improvement to their dexterity, learning to easily hold and play with toys

- Crawl and easily learn to go up and down a few stairs

- Eat well, are interested in food and enjoy mealtimes

Older children

- Are more creative

- Seem more emotionally balanced

- Can concentrate for longer

- Become better problem-solvers

- Are better able to make positive decisions

- Seem better able to learn and remember new things

- Often demonstrate a positive attitude to mealtimes and food

- Are more energetic during the day

- Are better able to create and maintain good relationships with others

And if your toddler or child is not sleeping well, then it goes without saying that you, as the parent, won't be sleeping either! According to America's Sleep Foundation, the average adult needs 7–9 hours of sleep every night. When you sleep only a few hours a night on an ongoing basis you build up a 'sleep debt' that can be hard to pay back. If your sleep debt persists over time then your health can seriously suffer.

ALISON SAYS . . .

'Sleep deprivation is recognized internationally as a form of torture! So why do we think it's OK that we don't sleep just because we have become parents? It will never make sense to me. I know that, given the right cues, nearly all babies and children are capable of sleeping soundly through the night.'

Typical sleep requirements

The sleep requirements of an individual baby, toddler or child can vary slightly, but the following table gives a general guide. This table will be useful to check the cumulative hours of sleep your little one is currently achieving and to better understand whether they are getting the required amount. Be aware that it's not just the cumulative sleep that's important; the sleep has to be established in line with the natural patterns of sleep.

For example, an eighteen-month-old who still has two day-time naps, doesn't go to sleep until 9 or 10pm, wakes once in the night and is up at 5am is definitely not following the natural rhythms of sleep and will most certainly be overtired.

0–5 years: typical sleep requirements per 24-hour period	
Newborn	16–18 hours
3 months	15–18 hours
6 months	15–17 hours
12 months	14–16 hours
2 years	14–15 hours
3 years	12–14 hours
4 years	11.5–12.5 hours
5 years	10.5–11.5 hours

Most children will still need a daytime nap until they are three years old. However, some toddlers give up their nap at two-and-a-half years old and others still enjoy one at nearly four. Whatever age, I advise some 'quiet-time', usually after lunch, around the same time that they would have been sleeping.

When to drop the daytime nap can cause a degree of uncertainty for parents. It's very difficult to say exactly when a toddler will be able to manage without a daytime nap, but there is more detailed information on how to assess this and how to implement quiet-time in later chapters.

Before addressing any sleep problem in your little one, it is important to look at their daily routine, well-being and health. Our sleep patterns are controlled by biological cycles, known as circadian rhythms, which repeat every 24 hours. These patterns of activity and rest affect digestion, body temperature and hormones, all of which need to keep a happy balance.

SLEEP CYCLES

There are two main types of sleep stage in newborn babies: rapid eye movement (REM), also known as 'active sleep', and non-rapid eye movement (NREM), also known as 'quiet sleep'. The different types of sleep last for periods known as 'sleep cycles' and are evident in your baby from birth. Newborns spend close to equal amounts of time in REM and NREM, but once babies reach around three months of age they begin to experience similar sleep cycles to adults, which comprise four distinct stages and are distinguished by different brain waves, as follows:

Sleep stages	Type of sleep	Normal length
Stage 1	NREM	1–5 minutes
Stage 2	NREM	10–60 minutes
Stage 3	NREM	20–40 minutes
Stage 4	REM	10–60 minutes

The first three stages of sleep are all NREM stages with the first two being lighter during which a person can easily be awakened. The third stage is the deepest and it is usually quite difficult to wake someone during this phase of sleep. REM is the fourth stage during which dreams can occur and adults will experience these stages in the order they are numbered.

At around five months of age the time spent in each cycle begins to mirror that of adult sleep, though babies will continue to have a short REM stage almost immediately after falling asleep instead of it being the last cycle, and this is why you will often notice your little one crying out or seeming to briefly wake a few minutes after falling asleep.

During REM sleep an infant's brain will be developing,

consolidating and solidifying various cognitive and physical skills. An adult's brain will be active in REM sleep too, and is when your mind processes the day's events and forms memories.

Generally, healthy adults sleep at least seven hours each night in a largely uninterrupted, single block of time. We have become used to our sleep patterns, with most of us unaware of the differing cycles through which we pass. However, babies have not yet learned the art of sleep and can be highly sensitive to their cycles. They will often wake after the first 40-minute cycle and struggle to go back to sleep, but by three months of age should have learned to self-soothe and easily drift off without intervention. However, I know many parents struggle with older babies who are still wakeful and seemingly unsettled throughout sleep.

Fortunately, understanding your child's sleep issue is the first step to resolving it. It's important to discover why and how things have become a problem, in order to implement an individually tailored plan that will bring positive change.

Sleep hygiene tips

- It's important to give your child regular exercise, but don't fall into the trap of thinking you need to wear them out every day, as this can cause overtiredness and make it harder for them to fall asleep.

- Daytime habits have an effect on sleep, so put in place a balanced daily schedule that includes periods of both rest and play.

- Provide a healthy and balanced diet, being mindful of any food intolerances.

- Establish and maintain a regular bedtime at the end of each day.

- Make the bedroom a no-screen zone, even during the day.

- Try to ensure the bedroom is kept quiet, and play some white noise to block out any excessive outside sounds.

- Keep the bedroom at a cooler temperature.

- Ensure the room is dark during the night; if needed, use blackout curtains to block any exterior light.

- Avoid giving sugary treats or dessert after 4pm and limit any snacks after dinner.

SLEEP DEPRIVATION AND ADHD

According to the Sleep Foundation, attention deficit hyper-activity disorder (ADHD) has become one of the most common conditions to be diagnosed during childhood, affecting approximately 3–5 per cent of school-age children and enduring throughout adolescence and into adulthood. It also states that cases of ADHD are increasing, and many parents with school-age children will be aware of a number of sufferers within their child's school and perhaps their classroom. No one can be certain whether more diagnoses are being made because there are more sufferers or because a better understanding of the condition is leading to more cases being identified.

The three main symptoms of ADHD in children and young people are:

- hyperactivity – the inability to sit still, as well as being fidgety, fiddling with things and suffering from sleep problems

- inattention – difficulty concentrating, being disorganized, forgetfulness and struggling to complete tasks

- impulsiveness – speaking out, acting without thinking, interrupting others and having difficulty waiting their turn

There is also now a proven link between sleep disorders (including sleep disruptions and deprivation) and ADHD. Numerous studies nearly all prove that a lack of sleep is a contributory factor and exacerbates ADHD symptoms. What remains unclear is whether sleep deprivation during a child's early months and years is a precursor to ADHD. A 2003 investigation by researchers at Tel Aviv University found that sleep deprivation resulted in a significant decrease in a child's ability to learn and sustain attention, and inhibited their emotional control. Interestingly, these are the three main areas of evaluation when diagnosing ADHD. We cannot state that sleep deprivation causes ADHD, but it massively contributes to the symptoms.

However, a report commissioned by the NHS, used as guidance for delivering effective services for children and young people with ADHD, barely mentions sleep. It gives clear advice and recommendations in many areas, but doesn't mention that the symptoms are exacerbated by a lack of sleep and therefore gives little advice on how to help and improve sleep issues.

ALISON SAYS . . .

'I truly believe that the link between ADHD symptoms and a lack of sleep is a very real concern and needs to be more fully addressed. Many of my clients also understand the seriousness of the situation and I have listened to many parents break down in tears when they confide to me that they have already been googling early-onset symptoms of ADHD and autism. They are often at the point of complete desperation as they witness their non-sleeping babies and toddlers become increasingly hyperactive and difficult to manage with each sleepless night that passes.'

I believe that health professionals' overriding focus should be on early intervention and improving sleep-quality in babies and children for the long term, but this doesn't seem to be the case. The NHS report only targets school-age children, which is too late given that studies suggest that improving sleep-quality within the first three years is of paramount importance for reducing the development of ADHD symptoms.

A PARENT'S STORY

'We called Alison to come and help with our baby boy, who wouldn't sleep at all or feed easily and who screamed the whole time. When Alison arrived, the first thing I did was to apologize to her in advance of meeting our three-year-old daughter, who was due home from nursery. Our daughter had been "difficult" from birth. Our doctors believed that she had some kind of ADHD. She often had severe tantrums that we couldn't control and it could take ages for her to calm down. She had been attending a special-needs nursery for a year. Although we had managed to get her to go to bed in the evening, she was always restless in sleep: thrashing about, sweating and crying out. I knew that she wasn't getting proper sleep, but I didn't know what to do. I was terrified our baby boy was going to follow the same path, which is why we asked Alison for help. When Alison met our little girl, she seemed to understand her immediately, having dealt with similar scenarios many times before. She explained what was causing all the tantrums and terrible behaviour: nearly everything stemmed from an undiagnosed acid-reflux problem and intolerances to dairy and wheat, which had made her so uncomfortable from birth that she was never able to sleep deeply. Since one month after implementing Alison's dietary changes and addressing the reflux, our little girl has been completely different. In fact, she is now the sweetest, kindest and most caring child you could ever meet. How different the first few years of her life could have been if we hadn't listened to those telling us we just had a bad sleeper and then the doctors telling us she was "on the spectrum". She clearly wasn't! We will always be eternally grateful to Alison, who literally changed our lives.'

E. D.

Throughout the following chapters there is further detail on all the topics mentioned above, along with information on many other contributing factors that can impact bedtime and sleep for your older baby or toddler. The book will give you explanations and advise how to manage different situations and implement changes.

☆ ALISON'S GOLDEN RULES ☆

1. Check the daily age-appropriate sleep requirements recommended for your child, using the chart in this chapter. They may need more sleep than you think!

2. Remember that children are designed to sleep and that no child is born to be a bad sleeper.

3. Understand that most children will respond positively to having a set routine with boundaries firmly in place.

4. Even if your toddler or child didn't sleep well as a baby, believe that by following my book things can change. It's never too late!

5. Ensure that you are providing the appropriate environment and atmosphere to promote healthy sleep associations.

6. Remember that toddlers and children can easily get overtired. You don't need to wear them out!

7. A daytime nap is still important for most children up to the age of three years.

8. Have faith that by following the methods set out in my book you can restore sleep to your household.

9. Know that you will need patience, and the older the child, the longer it can take for things to change. Consistency, patience and perseverance are key.

10. Implementing a new sleep schedule for your toddler can be challenging, so get support. It's much easier to do this with your partner or spouse by your side, or maybe there's another family member who can help. Ensure you've all read this book so everyone understands what to do and how to do it. Good luck!

CHAPTER 2

Toddler Development and Parenting Tips

An important part of being able to resolve your toddler's sleep issues is to understand the expected milestones that they should be reaching and the changes in their emotional, physical and cognitive development. This chapter includes invaluable information on why your toddler reacts in certain ways and what drives their behaviours, with tips to help you respond with positivity and confidence. There is also clear advice on how to implement boundaries and set routines, all of which underpin good sleep habits.

ALISON SAYS . . .

'Being a parent is the hardest and most important job in the world, yet one for which most of us have least training!'

DEVELOPMENTAL MILESTONES

'Developmental milestones' refer to specific skills that are reached at different stages. They fall into three main areas:

- cognitive milestones – reached through play, communication skills and learning

- physical milestones – as they discover how to crawl, stand up and walk

- emotional milestones – as they learn how to respond to others, control their emotions and follow instructions

Milestones your child will typically reach during the first three years will see them able to:

0–12 months	
• focus their vision • reach for toys • cuddle and kiss • smile and then giggle • wave and clap hands	• roll and then crawl • pull themselves up to standing and maybe take a first step • make sounds • develop bonds of trust
1–2 years	
• stand without support • walk unaided • participate in pretend play • develop speech, from sounds into words and then phrases • play simple ball games • follow simple instructions	• recognize themselves in a mirror or photograph • imitate behaviours of parents or other children • show greater independence • recognize and remember the names of familiar people

2–3 years	
• learn to run	• play games with other children
• stand on tiptoe	
• safely climb the stairs and come down	• go through a book one page at a time
• easily kick a ball	• express a wide range of emotions
• hold a crayon and scribble on paper	• speak in sentences
• sort objects by shape and colour	• recognize a few written words, including their name
• follow two- or three-step instructions	

This table is only a guide, however; all babies and toddlers reach their milestones at different times, contrary to what some books would have you believe. One popular book, *The Wonder Weeks*, states: 'All babies go through the same changes in mental development at the same time.'

While I agree that your baby, pre-toddler or toddler will experience many developmental changes during their first few years of life, I don't believe that these changes happen at exactly the same age in every child. In my experience, this ethos causes unnecessary stress in many parents, who worry that their baby is not reaching the stated milestones when expected, when there are so many things that will affect the development of a child and will have a bearing on when they reach certain milestones.

The Wonder Weeks also suggests that babies cry during developmental leaps as a reaction to undergoing such drastic change, and that 'being difficult' is therefore a sign that an amazing development has happened; little needs to be done as the baby will soon stop the bouts of crying. This leads to an acceptance that children's sleep may be disturbed for weeks at a time, and that toddlers will display poor behaviour and have tantrums, due to entering a developmental phase or due to sleep regressions. Instead, I believe that we should attempt to understand, assess and manage difficult behaviours or sleep issues instead of accepting them as the by-product of developmental phases.

As children develop, it can seem like everything you learned about your baby becomes redundant! Your relationship with them will need to evolve to match their ever-changing ways. They can seem to be changing almost daily at times, but then have periods where you will think they're regressing or not developing fast enough – toddlerhood can be a complete roller coaster and it can be a challenge to keep one step ahead of them!

It's important to be aware, however, that all toddlers take time to develop certain behavioural milestones compared with other developmental skills, in particular:

Emotional regulation There is a cluster of neurons in the brain primarily responsible for managing our emotions, called the amygdala. In relation to other milestones, the amygdala develops slowly in toddlers and is the main reason for their emotional outbursts.

Impulse regulation The prefrontal cortex of our brain is responsible for managing our impulse reactions and, like the amygdala, is underdeveloped in toddlers, which is why they often act on the spur of the moment, seemingly without thought or fear, and show immediate and over-the-top reactions to situations.

Being aware of this genuine lack of emotional and impulse control will hopefully make it easier to adapt your parenting methods and better understand your toddler's behaviour.

ALISON SAYS . . .

'On a recent phone consultation, a mum was telling me how upset she felt that her fourteen-month-old child was being labelled as aggressive. She felt he wasn't born that way and couldn't understand why he would bite her hand or pinch his grandma's leg, but then stroke the injured part and make an apologetic noise. It transpired that this little boy was in pain himself. He was suffering with acid-reflux, was intolerant to cow's milk and hardly slept because he was too uncomfortable. He didn't know how to express himself or ask for help and his "aggressive" behaviour was simply an unregulated impulsive act he carried out in response to the pain he felt inside. After two weeks of removing all dairy and soya from his diet, and with acid-reducing omeprazole prescribed by his GP, nearly all his "aggressive" behaviour had stopped.'

TODDLER GROWTH AND BEHAVIOURAL DEVELOPMENT

The early years are hugely important for establishing good health, and positive development in all areas will promote an all-round sense of well-being for the years ahead. Children's development happens in four key areas:

Cognitive development This refers to how children think, learn, acquire and retain knowledge, problem-solve and understand the world around them. There are four stages to cognitive development – reasoning, intelligence, language and memory – and while they all develop in infancy, you will see the most progression in toddlerhood.

Physical development This includes your toddler's growth as well as their gross and fine motor skills. (Gross motor skills require the use of larger muscles in the legs and arms; fine motor skills involve the use of smaller muscles in the fingers and hands.) While progression in this area will not be as pronounced or fast-changing for a toddler as it was in the infant stage, there will be many momentous developments.

Language development From twelve to thirty-six months, toddlers progress from using a handful of words to speaking in complete sentences. They will also learn to connect pictures with the objects, remember what things are called, recognize a written word and communicate more complex thoughts and ideas.

Social development This involves your toddler learning to adjust their behaviour to conform to societal expectations while also beginning to understand their own needs. They need to learn to ask for help, because it doesn't come naturally to them, and to learn to play and interact with others while developing a sense of self and independence.

All this growth and development may seem like a tall order for such a small child, but thankfully most of them take things in their stride and you will be amazed at the changes you see in them during these early years.

A PARENT'S STORY

'At twelve months my daughter started waking a couple of times in the night, having previously slept soundly for 12 hours. I researched this and believed it to be due to a developmental leap and therefore did nothing. I understood it would stop as soon as it started. Wrong! Over the next few weeks it got worse and worse, with multiple night-wakings, hours of screaming and even a complete bedtime refusal. It was awful and I couldn't understand how the leap had turned into this nightmare. I called Alison, and I'm so pleased that I did! She traced things back to when the problem started. We realized it wasn't linked to a leap at all, but due to me gradually introducing full-fat cow's milk as I weaned my daughter off breastfeeding. The national guidelines advice is to switch to ordinary cow's milk at twelve months and I had no clue that this was the root cause of my poor baby experiencing weeks of upset, tummy pain and stress. On Alison's advice, and after seeing a dietician, I switched to a plant-based milk and it was simply miraculous. Within three nights my daughter was back to enjoying bedtime and peacefully sleeping through the night.'

L.-M. D.

POSITIVE AND RESPONSIBLE PARENTING

How you respond to your toddler, along with the environment you provide for them, has a marked bearing on how they develop. While that may seem like a huge pressure, it doesn't need to be. If you can manage to adopt some of the following practices, they will promote a positive and healthy way forward.

- Have a daytime routine – not just a bedtime one. Children thrive on having a clearly defined sequence of steps, particularly for the challenging and chaotic parts of the day such as morning, getting dressed and breakfast.

- Establish healthy sleep habits. All of us need sleep, especially babies and young children.

- Ensure you have some quality one-to-one time. Toddlers thrive on attention, and providing some positive together time each day will bring huge benefits. For this to be effective, you really need to fully engage with your child: put your phone down, turn off the television and give them your undivided attention, even if it's just for a short time.

- Make your toddler feel included and give them a sense of responsibility. Toddlers need to have a sense of belonging, and encouraging them to contribute to daily chores teaches them that everyone, themselves included, is responsible for the smooth running of the home. The child who has everything done for them doesn't learn to respect their belongings, surroundings, or even themselves!

- Encourage your child to be a problem-solver. Watch her, talk to her, and calmly explain what she needs to do to resolve the frustration herself. This will encourage her to use her own skills to overcome challenges rather than relying on others to rescue her.

- Establish simple yet firm boundaries and household rules. Children respond more favourably when they understand what's allowed and what's not. All adults in the house need to be on the same page, so set up a clear framework of acceptable behaviours and provide a united approach when implementing and sticking to the rules.

- Be the 'responsible' parent and not just a nice one! It is my belief our children have a better chance of becoming balanced, well-rounded, responsible people themselves if we put boundaries and rules in place to guide them and keep them safe. Our children, toddlers and even babies *want* us to do this – they *like* knowing that you mean what you say, because this then means they can trust you. This means you need to be the person in charge, and that it's OK to have to say 'No' sometimes.

- Don't ignore the source of misbehaviour. Continual misbehaviour is nearly always a symptom of a deeper issue, and when you find what causes it you can use the right strategies to correct it. Is your child upset due to some changes, like starting nursery or feeling insecure after moving house? There are many life events that can have an effect on how your child behaves.

- Get outside! A change of scenery and some fresh air can bring some relief and alleviate the stresses of daily life. Try to have an outing once a day and enjoy the weather, be it sunshine, rain, wind or snow. Mother Nature provides us with an amazing backdrop to life wherever we live, and finding a puddle to jump in, some falling leaves to catch or some birds to watch brightens every day.

- Smile, laugh and have fun. I think this is almost the most important of all the above points – except, perhaps, for sleep! – as all aspects of life and parenting are much easier to deal with if we can adopt a happy and positive attitude. Life has a habit of throwing us challenges, and when things go awry we feel deflated, overtired, overworked or over-stressed. Smiling through it all and trying to find the funny side of life often seems to help. It also encourages our children to grow up with a positive outlook on life and to believe that we can overcome struggles, no matter what.

The following are other simple but important actions you can introduce to your daily or weekly routine that will help with your toddler's healthy development:

- Look at books with your little one and read to them daily. Books broaden your child's knowledge, and introducing them from a very young age can help with language and speech development. Teach your little one right from the start that books need to be looked after, not ripped, torn or drawn on.

- Talk to your toddler in your usual voice. Many parents, almost subconsciously, adopt a different tone when addressing their baby or toddler, which can cause some confusion for them.

- Engage your toddler to help with daily chores. Children love helping, and your child will learn so much from assisting you with the laundry, for example, as you explain what each item is or ask them to find the matching socks!

- Chat with your toddler and converse with them as much as possible to make them feel included. In the early years, 'conversations' may well be somewhat one-sided as you discuss what to cook for dinner, what you need to buy from the shops or who is coming for dinner at the weekend, but it all plays an important part in your child's speech- and language-development.

- Play matching games, sort shapes and do jigsaws. These simple activities help with cognitive development but are also fun and engaging ways of spending quality time with your little one.

- Listen to music with your toddler and sing with them. Music is known to help improve our mental health and boost endorphin levels, and though you may have music playing in the background during the day, set aside time just to have a singing and music session with your toddler. Along with the usual nursery rhymes, learn some songs together that involve actions, dance and sing-along, and listen to other types of music too.

- When out and about, or travelling in the car, devise simple games to play, such as 'Can you see a bus or a yellow car?' You could also play 'I spy' with colours before your little one can understand the word version (for example: 'I spy something red!'). You could collect leaves to take home and use glue and paper to make pictures with them, or find feathers and start a collection. You could keep a scrapbook or decorate a small box in which your child can put collected treasures like shells and pretty pebbles.

- Encourage your child's growing independence by letting him help to dress and feed himself. It's very tempting, especially when time is of the essence, to do these things yourself but, at less busy times, try to let them have a go.

- Try not to talk about your child in front of them. This is such a common and easy mistake. As adults, we wouldn't typically talk about someone else in front of them, as though they weren't in the room – it would be deemed rude and inappropriate. But parents do it all the time to their babies, toddlers and children, thinking it doesn't matter as the little ones don't understand. But they understand far more than you realize. They soak up everything being said about them, and even if they seem totally oblivious, they will still be listening. Remember – children have ears! It is far better to include your child in the conversation. For example, if you want to tell your husband, who has just returned from work, about something that your child did earlier in the day, have a conversation that includes your child and encourage them to take part in recounting the story.

A PARENT'S STORY

'When we got a new car, we paid extra to have screens in the back, thinking our two-year-old twins would benefit from watching DVDs on long journeys. The distraction certainly helped on the first couple of trips, but soon enough our little ones started demanding a film for every single outing in the car, even just to the shops. We had a few challenging weeks of tantrums if we didn't put the screens on, and if we turned it off while on the road they would both scream hysterically! It was awful and no journey was easy unless we bowed to their demands. Following Alison's advice, we put covers over the front seats that pulled down over the back, covering the screens, and explained to the twins that the screens were no longer working. Of course, we had huge tantrums at the start of the first outing, but they eventually calmed down. I then started the "Banana car" game that Alison had described. We all had to look for a yellow car and shout "Banana car!" when we saw one. The first yellow car caused so much excitement that the screens were soon forgotten. It was so much more enjoyable to be interacting with the girls on journeys! Thanks, Alison.'

K. P.

Encouraging good manners and respect

Manners need to be taught, shown and reinforced by parents and all caregivers who have authority within your child's life, and it's never too early to start. I believe that, in many ways, you can teach your child good manners from birth, and many of my clients have found it fascinating to witness my interaction with their little one when I'm working in their home. I always talk to the child, no matter what their age. I will 'discuss' things with them and vocalize their part in the 'conversation' by simply speaking for them, articulating what I would expect them to say in response.

You can do this yourself in any, or all, of the following ways:

- Talk to them as you're changing their nappy: 'Oops, sorry. Is that water too cold?'

- Ask them if they've had enough milk: 'Are you sure you don't want any more . . .? Aaah, you do: "Yes, please."'

- Engage with them throughout the day: 'Thank you – that was such a lovely little cuddle.'

- Vocalize their responses: 'Would you like to look at a book? Oh, yes, please, that would be lovely. OK, come on then.'

- Converse with them at mealtimes: 'Would you like a drink of water now? OK, no thank you, perhaps in a minute.'

I know many parents have secretly thought me a bit mad (and maybe I am!), but I know this sort of talk really promotes wonderful manners in the longer term. The National Literacy Trust agree: they believe that talking to your child from birth is the foundation of vocabulary, literacy and even positive mental health, and they provide numerous resources and tips on how to 'talk to your baby'.

If you want your little angel to grow up with angelic manners then you need to use them too. A toddler who grows up hearing polite and respectful language within the home will most likely follow that example.

To teach and reinforce good manners, start with 'please' and 'thank you'. Be consistent and use the words each time it is appropriate, also vocalizing them for your toddler when it's the appropriate response. Once they are able to make sounds or form words, you can encourage them to respond themselves instead of speaking for them.

Baby and toddler signing became very popular a number of years ago and is hugely beneficial as children can usually learn a sign and use it before they can speak the word.

Over the years, I've attended many different social activity classes with various families and I've always endorsed 'sing and sign' sessions. I love the concept of combining music with learning, and these classes also promote the use of good manners and respectful behaviour, as some of the first signs that children learn are for 'please', 'thank you', 'hello' and 'goodbye' (as well as signs for 'happy', 'sad', 'cry', 'laugh' and 'love').

The use of 'hello' and 'goodbye' will already be understood by your toddler by the time she is around twelve months old, and she will likely be waving to family members as they come and go. As your child gets older, developing good manners for arrivals and departures can become more challenging: though you might expect your toddler to greet people at the door and politely say goodbye to them when they leave, this may not be the reality. Toddlers can find it tricky to adapt when someone arrives at their home and it can take them a while to adjust, but they usually open up and start chatting to the visitor soon enough. If your toddler is refusing to say 'Hello' when someone arrives, don't try to force it. It can be helpful to prepare your toddler if you know someone is calling round to see you, by telling her 'Auntie Lucy is coming to see us today. It will be lovely to see her and we can give her a big welcome when she arrives.' This will give your little one time to mentally adjust and hopefully promote a happy and polite greeting.

Another good way to encourage good manners is through mealtimes and sitting together at the table. It can be a major achievement for some toddlers to learn to sit still and I often feel it's unfair to expect them to stay at the table when eating alone. Where possible, try to sit with your toddler through mealtimes and eat with them. When your child is about to throw some food on the floor, you can put out your hand and ask them to give it you if they don't want it, saying 'thank you' as they do so. Establish good table manners by explaining that we all sit and wait for everyone to finish, or that your family says prayers and blesses the food before eating. Of course, adding in and encouraging the appropriate use of 'please' and 'thank you' throughout mealtimes will pay dividends, and your heart will swell with pride when your child independently says 'Thank you' to the waiting staff on an outing to a restaurant.

Setting boundaries

For their own well-being, it is really important that children have, and understand, boundaries. Setting limits in order to encourage good habits is just as essential as love and hugs.

I've visited many homes where the child or children seem to be ruling the roost, with no set bedtime and dictating to their parents what they want and when they want it! If this is a situation you are happy with, then that is absolutely fine and it is totally your choice, but mostly the parents of such children are desperate to know how to find some structure and ask me for guidance on how to set boundaries to create a more harmonious home environment.

Before you set the boundaries or 'house rules', you have to decide what they are going to be. I actively encourage parents to discuss their parenting plans and beliefs with each other from the outset. This way you can devise your parental strategies together and agree a framework from which to move forward.

The easy-to-follow strategies below will allow you to create and set boundaries that your children will understand.

Set clear expectations

Once you have decided what your 'house rules' are going to be, prioritize those that are most important. It's better to start off with just a few basic rules and introduce others as necessary. Make sure you are clear when giving instructions and remain unified in your approach. It's very important that both parents, as well as any other adults providing care for your children, implement the same house rules and in the same manner.

Some suggestions for your basic rules:

- Be kind and gentle – no hurting anyone

- Shoes off at the front door

- No climbing on the furniture

- Use nice words and don't shout

- Listen to one another

- Sit at the table to eat

- Look after our things

Start early

Many parents mistakenly think that babies and toddlers are too young to understand and they therefore don't stop or correct irritating or bad behaviours. These can soon develop into habitual behaviours that are harder to stop or change, so it's better not to let them develop in the first place.

Implement safety guidelines that are set in stone

These are important rules that you need to have in place to keep your child safe at all times, inside and outside the home. For example:

- Always hold a caregiver's hand when crossing the road

- Always wear a seatbelt in the car

- Never play with scissors or sharp knives

- Never run on a slippery floor

- Never touch the hot-water tap or a hot drink

- Never run off or go out of sight

- Never speak with strangers

It is important to always explain why you want them to follow these rules, in a manner that they can understand.

Be a good role model

There was a parenting phrase coined many years ago and I can still hear my father saying it: 'Don't do as I do, do as I say!' The trouble with this ethos is that children learn by imitating and copying your behaviour, so it is much better for you, as parents, to display the behaviours you want your little ones to adopt. For example, if you want your children to learn that interrupting someone while they are speaking is unacceptable, then try not to interrupt others or your children when they are talking. Many of the boundaries you want to set in place can be implemented simply by demonstrating them yourself. When in the car, you could say, 'I'm buckling my seatbelt because it keeps me safe', or when arriving home you might say, 'I'm taking my shoes off at the front door because they are dirty'. Acting out and explaining your behaviour is such a simple but effective way of showing your child the rules you want your household to live by.

Be consistent

Whatever rules or boundaries you are trying to set, it is important to demonstrate consistency and keep the rules in place every day. Avoid creating confusion by relaxing the rules one day and then reinstating them the next. Your toddler simply will not understand them if he's allowed to climb on the table one day, but told to get down the next.

Time management

If you can teach your child the value of time, habits like punctuality and good time management can become ingrained from a young age. However, children have little concept of time, so when you tell your toddler to come to the table in ten minutes, they don't know how long that will be. In certain situations you could use a timer or an alarm on your smartphone – for example, to give a warning that it is nearly time to leave the park. Once children can read numbers, you can use a digital clock, explaining that it will be snack time when a ten appears. As they begin to comprehend a clockface, you can teach them how to identify 5- or 10-minute sections and use them as time warnings.

Offer healthy choices

Toddlers are always looking for ways to be independent, which is why they sometimes will 'push back' and resist boundaries or rules. It can help your child to accept boundaries if you can give them some choice in other areas – for example, which plate to use for lunch, what colour socks to wear, or the blue or yellow cup for a drink. However, toddlers' brains are not yet developed enough to make important or complex decisions, so keep the choices you give simple, offering no more than two options at a time. For instance, most young children will change their minds often, and if you ask them whether they want fish, pasta or an omelet for lunch, by the time you cook and serve their requested option they may decide they want one of the other choices and be disappointed that you followed their initial instructions!

Don't allow situations to escalate

Toddlers will often make demands that you need to refuse, and this can easily escalate into conflict. When a requested item is not forthcoming, your child may quickly collapse into a sobbing heap and become irrational. This is normal toddler behaviour, as their impulse and emotional reactions are not yet regulated, and it can be tricky to manage the situation.

Firstly, consider carefully what your child is asking for. If you are happy for her to have the requested chocolate bar, let her know that she can have it because you've decided she can have it. You could say something like 'I've had a little think and because you helped me so nicely this morning, yes, you can have the treat.' It's important for your child to understand that you're not just saying 'yes' because she demanded the chocolate, but more because you're in control of giving the treat.

However, if you feel it is inappropriate to say 'yes' and you do not want her to have the requested chocolate bar, then you have to stick to your guns – do not give in after a period of time. I advise what I call the 'three-strike rule'; the answer will be 'no' but there's a simple but effective way of saying this:

1. **First, you politely say 'no' but also give an explanation for this.**
   Avoid saying 'no' for the sake of it; it's really important to explain why you aren't giving the treat at this time. Unfortunately this doesn't necessarily mean that requests for the item will stop, and any continuing demands will lead you into the second strike.

2. **If the request is repeated, you reiterate that the answer is 'no' and refer back to the explanation you've already given.**
   This is a firm reminder that you've already said no and why this is, which gives her the opportunity to back down, realize you mean what you say and accept your decision on the matter. However, if the protests and demands escalate, you will need to respond by using strike three.

3. **If your toddler asks again, stand firm with the answer of 'no', remind her you've already explained twice and that you're not going to tell her again, and that the matter is now closed.** This will be your final say on the matter. If the protests turn into a full-blown tantrum, try to ignore her and do not mention the topic again. The more you talk about it and try to reason with her, the more you fuel the situation, so try to just use some distraction techniques and soon enough it will all be forgotten.

See promises and consequences through

I have heard many parents making idle threats to their toddler that they don't see through or act upon. A classic and commonly used one is at mealtimes, when the toddler is told they will not get pudding if they don't eat their main course – and yet, despite consuming very little of their main course, pudding appears! It is equally easy to make other commitments to your little one, such as promising to play a game or read a book, that are then not delivered because you run out of time, for example. None of these scenarios are created by parents who are intentionally malicious or overindulgent, but they are unfair and will have a negative impact on how your child behaves and responds. A toddler will learn that you don't mean what you say, and over time they will find it hard to take any of your bargaining seriously, as they simply won't believe you'll follow through. The bond of trust that should blossom and grow between parent and child will instead become somewhat fractured, which in turn leads to a lack of parental control.

Similarly, if you're going to issue a consequence for unacceptable behaviour, you have to mean it and go through with it. In the heat of the moment, when trying to manage your toddler in full tantrum, you might say something like 'If you do that again then you're not going to go swimming' – yet even though they do the same thing, again and again, they still get to go swimming later that day. I understand it's often easier to 'give in' as you may have arranged to meet friends there or simply because it is a lesson you've paid for and don't want to miss, but the point here is not to make an idle threat, because your toddler will quickly learn that you don't mean what you say. This can also have a knock-on effect if your child starts not to trust other things you say, such as promises, commitments or even information and advice.

Once a child understands that you mean what you say, life will be much easier to manage.

Praise your child

This is a simple and natural way to endorse your child's positive behaviour, but there are some subtle tips to keep in mind. Simple approvals such as 'Well done for listening', 'You're so clever for getting dressed by yourself', 'You're so kind for giving your sister her toy' and 'You're so helpful – thank you for tidying up your books' are easy ways to give positive praise throughout the day.

However, it is easy to give too much praise in certain scenarios and inadvertently create too much hype around normal life experiences and transitions. Learning to use the toilet is a classic example. The first time a toddler does a wee in the potty, everyone claps, cheers and bestows so much praise on her that she may feel confused and overwhelmed. After all, it's likely that she has witnessed you using the toilet on a daily basis without everyone saying how clever you are! In this situation, compliment at a slightly lower level, without an unnecessary, over-the-top celebration. This will help to normalize the act of going to the loo – which, after all, is something we do multiple times a day – and prevent it from becoming a high-pressure task and one that she knows will gain her attention.

Also, give praise when they least expect it. When your toddler is sitting playing with some toys on her own, it is tempting to leave her to it and get on with household chores. While it is important that your little one has this alone-time to develop her imagination and independence, it is also important to recognize that she has been playing nicely and to praise her for it. All too often, more attention is given when a child is acting in an unacceptable way. This fuels them to act up, as they learn that they get more attention for negative behaviour.

A PARENT'S STORY

'When my little girl was three, she loved to sit on her beanbag and look through her books. I would often leave her and not interfere, but I would always comment on how nicely she treated her books and how pleased it made me to see her happy and enjoying them. I would also engage with her and ask her a question about one or two of the books that she had looked at, so that she knew that I was watching and had an interest in her activity. One day, when she received a new book as a present for her eighth birthday, she turned to me and said, "I remember when I was little, I used to sit on my beanbag and look at my books, and I was always surprised when you would talk to me afterwards, as I didn't know you were watching me. It's one of my happiest memories." I was so proud to know that the unexpected praise and interest that I had offered back then has turned into a long-term, happy memory for my daughter.'

J. H.

Focus on the behaviour, not the child

If you need to correct or address the way your child is acting, try to comment on what the child is doing, rather than the child themselves. Instead of saying, 'You're so naughty to do that', it is much better to say something like, 'I'm disappointed with that behaviour; I really hope it won't happen again.' This separates your child from the negative behaviour and teaches them that it's OK to make mistakes, we all do, but that it's important to learn from them and to try to avoid the disappointing behaviour.

Be direct with your requests

So many parents make the mistake of *asking* their child to do something instead of *telling* them, which creates an opportunity for conflict to arise. If you need your child to put on his shoes because you are going outside, say, 'It's time to put your shoes on now,' rather than asking, 'Shall we go and put on our shoes?' A question only opens the door for your child to immediately respond with 'No.' Quite why children answer with a 'no' so often is something of a mystery, but they usually do!

SOCIALIZING AND LEARNING TO SHARE

Social interaction will help your toddler to develop a sense of self and to achieve significant developmental breakthroughs. It will also allow him to become familiar with social expectations that others may have of him. Getting your child to socialize is not always easy, but there are a few healthy habits that can be established from an early age, such as learning to share and to resolve conflict, that will promote positive behaviour when he is among other children and become skills for life.

Playdates

A good way of promoting pleasant manners, social graces and respect is through regular playdates. There can be tricky moments, of course – there are often quarrels over toys, perhaps your toddler doesn't want to share, or maybe they won't join in at all and go off to sulk! But while you may sometimes need to intervene and help solve the problem, it's important to try to find the balance and sometimes allow the children to work things out for themselves.

The best way to ensure that playdates with young children run smoothly is to set the rules and boundaries beforehand, with all adults in agreement. However, while this sounds sensible, it can be difficult to implement as there isn't always unity and openness between parents of young children. I've witnessed parents dreading playdates with certain other toddlers because they always end in chaos, with broken toys, injuries and squabbles. Often the hosting parent is reluctant to intervene and manage the visiting child's behaviour, for fear of upsetting the other parent.

It can be really difficult to have an open and honest discussion with another parent about parenting strategies for a playdate and many feel quite anxious at the thought of initiating any such conversation. However, a joint parenting plan to use when socializing your children would be hugely beneficial. Here are some suggestions and questions you could pose:

- Let's make sure the children say 'please' and 'thank you'.

- We'll put away your toddler's special or precious toys before the playdate.

- We can explain to the children that we will use a 10-minute timer to ensure they each get a turn on the tractor or bike.

- If there's a continuing argument over a specific toy, let's agree to remove it from the room completely.

- Please could we make sure the children sit down for their snack, as that's the rule we always have in our house.

- How shall we manage any aggressive or harmful behaviour, like biting or kicking?

- We don't let our children climb on the furniture and your toddler is a bit of a mountaineer! Is it OK to keep our rule in place when you come over and to dissuade any climbing inside?

- Can we agree that the children tidy everything away after the playdate?

If you can be brave and find the strength to open the discussion about managing toddler behaviour on any playdates or social outings, it will create a much happier and more peaceful experience for you, your toddler and the other families involved.

Sharing

Toddlers don't understand the concept of sharing and it takes some time for them to learn this art. At the age of eighteen months they are just getting to grips with understanding that they have 'belongings' – lovely toys and beautiful books, which have been given just to them. All of sudden, we then expect them to share their things with a visiting toddler. It's no wonder this 'horror' can induce extreme reactions, but don't panic, they are not being selfish; it is natural for them to be possessive over their toys, and even of you! Indeed, 'my' and 'mine' are some of the first words a toddler will learn to use when claiming ownership of an object. This actually reflects a very clever developmental phase in which he is grasping the abstract concept of a person's invisible tie to a 'thing'. Some research suggests that children between the ages of two and four tend to believe that the person who possesses an object first is the rightful owner, even if someone else gets hold of it later. This also explains why they may go through the phase of unequivocally believing that you, as their parents, belong to them! The statement 'I had it first' would certainly be a strong argument in a toddler-led court of law!

Here are some simple strategies you can implement to encourage your little one to learn how to share, borrow and return.

- Share something of your own with your child. Explain that the item belongs to you but that you're happy to share it with them.

- Let them borrow something that is yours. Make sure they are aware that they can have it for a short while and then must give it back.

- Let them have some 'special' items, which they don't have to share and are put away before visitors arrive. Explain that other people have 'special' items that we mustn't touch when we go to their house.

- Don't tell them off when they don't share. Instead, try to validate their feelings and give the other child something else to play with.

- Take them to the library, as it is not only a fabulous resource, but also helps to explain the concept of borrowing, looking after items that belong to someone else and then returning them.

TECHNOLOGY AND SCREEN TIME

Smartphones and screens have become an integral part of our lives, and it's almost impossible to keep them away from children. Tablets can provide a wonderful learning resource for young children, as well as entertainment, but left with unrestricted access children can quickly become addicted to screens and could happily spend hours on them. Equally, they will often be reluctant to give them up unless they have learned from the start that they only have access at certain times.

Parents have worried about how much time children spend in front of screens for the past fifty years, ever since television became an accepted part of life. A survey conducted in the late 1950s found that 5.7 million homes owned a television set, which was about one in three, but by the late 1970s, 93 per cent of homes had their own TV. Interestingly, the number of homes that own a television has decreased throughout the past decade as more people are watching programmes on their laptops, tablets and smartphones.

In most homes today there are a multitude of media inlets. Often, each room in the house has a screen of some description, so children grow up seeing screens and online access as a normal part of life. However, I believe it is important to limit and supervise screen time for young children, just as I said twenty years ago to parents who asked if it was OK to let their little ones watch television. I have always said that all television viewing should be under parental supervision and that children should not have free access to watch whatever they choose, whenever they want, and I think the same principle is best adopted for all types of screen time today.

Toddlers do not *need* televisions, screens or tablets, and have developed without them since time began. I think we would all agree that engagement in the physical world, quality one-to-one attention and getting outside for exercise in the fresh air are far preferable ways for your child to learn. Nonetheless, we have to accept that screens and technology are here to stay. With that in mind, there are a number of issues to consider that will help you control their use:

Encouraging a shared experience

As with books, the benefit of a shared viewing experience with an adult is often a far healthier learning and emotional experience for your child. Admittedly, it's hard to resist the temptation to turn on the television or plonk your toddler in front of a screen, knowing they will sit quietly for some time engrossed in a cartoon. But while this can occasionally be a useful tool to allow you some much-needed space, it's also important to have times when you engage with your little one throughout their screen use. Perhaps you might allow your child a timed session, where he can sit and watch one or two cartoon episodes for the same duration each day, whereas at other times you will engage with him in either watching something or playing a screen-based game together.

Regulating instant gratification

Many simple games and apps that children use give virtual rewards like coins or sweets, which bring a sense of instant gratification to your toddler. In turn, this will give her brain a dopamine boost, which leads to an addictive desire to continue to play the game. Dopamine is a hormone released in the brain in response to feeling a sense of gratification, and it plays a major role in the motivational part of reward-motivated behaviour. This is why young children can so easily become obsessed with playing these games, so be prepared to implement some firm parenting to keep screen access to the desired level.

Open access to all life events

Before smartphones and social media, we would often learn of life events only through a landline telephone call or by post. Today we are constantly receiving messages, social media posts and online news, some of which might upset us. If we're in front of our children when we react badly – for example, if you read some upsetting news just as you have sat down to lunch with your toddler – they will witness your sharp intake of breath, your tears or your anger, and this response will cause them to feel upset too. While children need to learn about life events and how to cope with them, avoiding such messages until you are in private, or while your toddler is sleeping, at least gives you time to compose yourself and to prepare what to tell your little one – if, indeed, they even need to know what has happened.

Technoference

This is a new term to describe the growing phenomenon of smartphone obsession. More than 5 billion people worldwide are now estimated to own a mobile device. A quick scroll through Instagram or a hastily written response to an email or text might not seem like a big deal, but the most important thing for children aged under three is interaction with human beings, and anything that disrupts or interferes with the timing, meaningfulness or emotional quality of that interaction can have consequences for the relationship between parents and their children. However, technology can be an incredibly helpful tool for parents, with online parent forums, instant information access, feeding-tracker apps and high-quality educational apps for children, so it definitely has a place. Still, most experts agree that when it comes to infants and toddlers, it's best to avoid or severely restrict your own screen use when with them.

Parental guilt

Many researchers agree that recent developments within Western culture have cultivated an idealized expectation that all parents should be caring, nurturing, patient and, above all else, ever-present. This guilt-inducing ethos of perfectionism can also be referred to as the 'goddess mother myth' and can cause unnecessary stress and pressure for parents, and particularly mothers, who feel they must be perfect. One area that fuels this parental guilt is allowing your little ones to use screens. Many parents will hand over a mobile phone to distract their upset toddler while sitting in a waiting room or so they can get things done around the home, but then feel guilty about it, especially if they feel the disapproving gaze of others when they do it. To avoid these feelings of guilt building up, devise a set plan to determine when you will allow screen time and when you won't. Then *stick to it* and feel confident about your boundaries.

Blue light and bedtime

The blue light present in sunlight boosts our attention, memory, energy levels, reaction times and overall mood. It's the signal to our brains that we should be up and about and active. At night, meanwhile, the absence of blue light from the sun tells us that we should be resting. The problem these days is that we are surrounded by artificial sources of blue light – particularly from the screens on our electronic devices – that confuse these signals. Blue light at night suppresses the release of melatonin in our brains needed for good-quality sleep, which is why it is really important to avoid screen time for your toddler or child for at least two hours before bedtime. I know many parents rely on using a screen to distract a toddler when dealing with a new baby, for example, but try using books or audiobooks instead.

Parental supervision, authorization and control

Whatever access to screens you decide to allow, it is vital that your child is protected and safe, and that they are only viewing content that has been deemed suitable for their age by the regulating authority. You also don't want them to run up high costs by accidentally downloading apps or add-ons without your knowledge. There are many ways of keeping your little one safe online, whether by using an account linked to your own that requests your permission before any content is downloaded, along with other specific permission settings, or by using a specifically designed safeguarding app. Until children are much older, I believe it is also best to keep television remote controls out of reach so that children don't have instant access.

A PARENT'S STORY

'We had welcomed our third baby three months earlier and Alison was staying with our family to introduce a bedtime routine, just as she had with our first two, who were now four and two years old. Completely out of the blue, our four-year-old started crying at bedtime, saying he didn't like the dark and wanted a light on. We put a night-light on but he still wouldn't sleep until exhaustion overtook him. This carried on for three more nights and we were perplexed by this sudden change in behaviour. The next day we had to take the baby to see a doctor and Alison came with me, sitting in the back of our car with the baby in a car seat. As I drove off, the car's DVD player came on. I was about to turn it off when Alison said to let it play as it directly related to our son's bedtime. It was an episode of *Dora the Explorer* and in the cartoon Dora was on a train that had stopped at a tunnel and refused to go in. The train was saying it was scared of the dark! A few days before, my son had been watching this episode in the back of the car and I hadn't realized what it was about. It was obvious that this was the cause of his fear at bedtime and he was just imitating the behaviour he had witnessed on the screen! After that, I always tried to watch any programmes before I let the children view them.'

C. R.

Positive and responsible parenting takes time and patience, and it can be challenging to implement it 24/7, so focus on the basics and celebrate your successes. Try not to feel guilty about the times when you run out of steam, lose your patience or even shout at your toddler. Take a deep breath, have a cup of tea (or look forward to something stronger later that evening) and know that you are an amazing parent, you're only human, none of us is perfect and your little one will survive your temporary loss of control.

☆ ALISON'S GOLDEN RULES ☆

1. Try not to worry about 'getting it all right' or being the 'perfect parent' – you are more than good enough! Have faith in yourself, celebrate the things that feel good and don't focus on the times when it all goes awry.

2. Children thrive when being praised with endorsements. If they experience negativity and criticism, they will grow up with low self-esteem.

3. Use direct instructions when you need your toddler to do something. It's OK to tell them what they need to do and when you want them to do it!

4. Try to reinforce manners by being polite, considerate and showing respect yourself.

5. Devise and set your boundaries and house rules from the start. It's never too early for your child to learn right from wrong.

6. Remember that positive and responsible parenting takes effort. Try not to give in or take the path of least resistance on every occasion. Stick to your guns and mean what you say.

7. Allow your child the space to develop a sense of independence and to learn from their mistakes.

8. Be brave and discuss parenting tactics with other parents when socializing your little ones.

9. Keep control of any devices. It's much easier to have boundaries from the start rather than to curtail any previously-allowed freedoms.

10. Remember that parenting is much easier when your toddler is well-rested and getting their full quota of sleep. Follow all the steps in this book to give the whole family a full night's rest and enjoy peaceful nights for years to come.

CHAPTER 3

Developmental Changes and Sleep

Sleep for babies and children can be fraught with challenges and obstacles, including many factors that manifest as babies get older. This chapter will give you information that may be key to understanding why your older baby or toddler may not be sleeping – from environmental factors to possible causes of bedtime fears or night terrors. It will also detail just how much sleep is needed according to your child's age, along with suggested schedules and routines, including daytime naps or 'quiet-time' once daytime sleep is no longer required. I'll also be giving you my view on the infamous 'sleep regressions', a research-based explanation of the term 'sleep-training', and some information on the little-understood but crucial 'forbidden sleep zone'.

GENETICS AND ENVIRONMENTAL INFLUENCES

Children come in different shapes and sizes and each has their own personality, with no two children ever the same – even identical twins have differences in personalities.

Among the factors that will influence your child's personality are birth order and growing up with one or more siblings who have come before or after them, so even siblings raised by the same parents, living in the same home, will grow up in somewhat different environments.

There are also many variations in parental circumstances that will also have an effect on how your child develops. The range of parental configurations is vast, with some examples being:

- older parents

- younger parents

- parents in a heterosexual relationship

- same-sex couples

- single parents

- estranged mothers or fathers

- blended families

- parents from different cultures

- parents from different religions

- working parents

- stay-at-home parents

- parents who frequently move house or travel a lot

What's more, all parents have different personalities, along with their own unique life experiences that will also shape their parenting styles and contribute to the evolving environment in which a child grows up.

We also need to consider the genetics of each child – their DNA and how that has been created – as this, too, will have an effect on their development. Interestingly, in the past few decades there has been much research into epigenetics – how the environment can change the make-up of your DNA. This includes research carried out by the Center on the Developing Child at Harvard University which showed that environmental influences and children's experiences affect the way their genes develop. During early-years development, the DNA that makes up our genes accumulates chemical markers or imprints, together known as the 'epigenome', which determine how much or little of the gene is expressed. This explains why genetically identical twins can develop different behaviours and why their skill-sets vary, with their health and cognitive development differing too.

The research found that the epigenome can be affected by both positive experiences – such as loving homes, supportive relationships and engaged learning – and negative ones – like an unhealthy environment, emotional abuse and stressful life circumstances; they all leave a unique epigenetic signature, or mark, on the DNA, which affects how the genes develop. This means that the old idea that genes are 'set in stone' has been disproven and that 'nature versus nurture' is no longer a debate – the answer is it's nearly always both!

Young brains are very sensitive to epigenetic changes. With your toddler's brain developing so rapidly, their experiences in these early years have a huge impact and can cause epigenetic adaptations that influence when and how their genes release instructions that will influence their future health, skills and resilience. That's why it's crucial to provide supportive and nurturing experiences, along with good sleep health, for children in the earliest years.

We know that sleep deprivation leads to increased stress levels in many babies and children, so for children who are constantly overtired and therefore suffering from stressful living experiences, the effect of the epigenetic marks on the DNA may be a more negative one.

However, while we now know all about the epigenetics and how the environment and life experiences can affect a child's development, it's also important to understand that, although negative experiences may leave an imprint on the genes, the imprint can be lessened and somewhat 'wiped off' by ensuring there are more positive experiences that follow.

At various times in our lives, many of us have to face difficult problems, deal with negative situations, manage traumatic life events or work through previous childhood issues. Coping during these tough periods can be extremely challenging for us all, but even more so when we are managing parenthood at the same time. The natural, parental instinct is to shield and protect our children from our ordeals; we may think that in an ideal world they should never have to know about any family problem or see their parents upset or angry. But that's simply not the reality and almost impossible to achieve. I believe it is also important for young children to learn that the reality of life is that it's not always without problems. If they grow up having been completely shielded and almost living in a protective bubble, they will be less equipped to deal with the challenging situations they will face as they grow up.

So, when you feel your parenting is somewhat lacking and you're managing a difficult time in life, don't be too hard on yourself. Ditch the guilt, take off the pressure and do what you need to get through. Your child will be absolutely fine!

ALISON SAYS . . .

'I have stayed with thousands of families over the years, and I can truly say that there isn't one home that I've left and thought, "Wow, they have the perfect life, are the perfect parents and have the perfect children." Perfection simply doesn't exist! I applaud you all.'

CAN SLEEP DISORDERS BE HEREDITARY?

Many times I have heard parents talk about their own sleep issues and relate them to their child's seeming inability to sleep, but just because you might not sleep well yourself, it doesn't necessarily follow that your child should suffer the same problem.

Research has shown there are only four sleep disorders that have a proven genetic basis:

- fatal familial insomnia

- familial advanced sleep-phase syndrome

- chronic primary insomnia

- narcolepsy

All of these conditions are quite rare, so most sleep problems in babies and children will not have been passed down through genetics or be in any way truly hereditary. Instead, they will mostly be linked to a child's experiences and environment – the epigenetic influences I described earlier in this chapter.

However, it's almost certain that a parent's anxiety and high stress levels surrounding sleep will often contribute to, or be the whole cause of, the reason a child is not sleeping. Sadly, I've found this to be the case with many parents who have described their own negative associations with sleep. Examples of such scenarios in adults are:

- feeling fear as a child and not wanting to be alone or go to bed

- hearing parental arguments downstairs while they were in bed, as a child

- being bullied as a child, which induced such stress that it affected their sleep

- seeing an inappropriate film as a youngster, which sparked off a night-time fear

- hearing one of their parents talk about their own sleep problems, which caused them to adopt a sleep issue themselves

- suffering some kind of childhood trauma, which resulted in them being terrified of the dark or night-time in general

- experiencing high stress levels and pressure at university or at work, leading to insomnia

- undergoing a life-changing or life-threatening event, since which they have never slept properly

There are so many reasons that sleep has been, or can become, an issue, and try as you might to hide these fears or associations when becoming parents, it's actually incredibly difficult to do so and can simply increase any concern that you have 'caused' your little one's sleep issues or 'passed on' your own anxieties surrounding sleep. But as many of my clients already know, these associations can be halted and turned around fairly easily.

A PARENT'S STORY

'My biggest fear when I was pregnant was that I would pass on my awful sleep habits to my baby. My phobia around sleep started when I heard my parents fighting downstairs; I just lay there awake in bed, frozen with fear.

Soon after that, my parents split up and my father left, and although life became OK in many ways, I always hated going to bed and would just lie awake for hours. Fast-forward to adulthood, and I still carried with me an innate fear of bedtime; add on the pressures and stress of work and I rarely had a good night's sleep.

I found Alison's book and was fully prepared to implement her newborn sleep routine, believing my baby would learn to love sleep by following "The Plan". However, no one prepared me for how I would feel when my baby actually arrived, and due to the huge pressure I felt at becoming a mum, my anxieties about sleep started to soar. I became obsessed with my baby's napping and night-time sleep, and when she didn't sleep I would just panic. In hindsight, I realize that my worries created such a tense atmosphere; I would constantly check her to see if she was still asleep.

I battled on for months, eventually believing that I had passed on my fears to my baby and that she would hate sleep as much as I did. When my daughter was fourteen months old, Alison came to stay and completely turned things around. She helped me access support to deal with my anxiety and undiagnosed post-natal depression. She "removed" me from all sleep-associated situations with my daughter and worked with my partner on implementing the sleep-training my daughter needed.

Once my daughter was sleeping as she should, I felt an immediate sense of relief and, over time, my fears subsided as I believed my daughter could actually sleep! Of course, I found it difficult when I had to take back control and was in charge of her nap and bedtimes again, but it was so much easier as I knew she could do it.'

H. T.-J.

SLEEP-TRAINING

In scientific literature 'sleep-training' is an umbrella term that refers to a spectrum of approaches that help babies learn to fall asleep by themselves. There is a wide variety of techniques, ranging from gradual withdrawal, where you give less and less physical contact and presence over a number of weeks, to a continual 'pick up and put down' approach through to a complete 'cry-it-out' method. Unfortunately, the latter seems to have become synonymous with any use of the phrase 'sleep-training' and whenever the term is used people immediately assume you are leaving your baby to cry themselves to sleep. As a result, sleep-training has become an extremely emotive subject and a hotly debated topic within the parenting world. Even the mention of 'sleep-training' can induce an angered response from some.

The advocates and opponents have set up their camp on each side of the divide, with seemingly no middle ground. Proponents argue that it does not harm the baby and has benefits for both the child and their family. Opponents focus only on 'cry-it-out' techniques, saying they are cruel to children and cause long-term problems. Unfortunately, much of the debate is fuelled by misinformation, which is sad and unnecessary since there is actually a great deal known about children's sleep and much can be learned from the scientific studies.

The saying 'It takes a village to raise a child' is so true. Throughout most of human history, children have typically been raised within large and extended family units. However, in today's society many parents are almost 'going it alone' without much help at all, and trying to find the time to implement and establish positive sleep associations from the outset can be incredibly tiring. Understandably, many parents will take the path of least resistance and just let their baby sleep on them the whole time. But a few weeks, months or even years later comes the realization that they can't put their child down at all and that no one is getting much sleep. Only at this point do they decide to implement some form of 'sleep-training' to teach their little one how to fall and stay asleep on their own.

Following my own research and over twenty years' experience of working with babies, toddlers and children, I devised my own method, my hugely successful reassurance sleep-training technique. It is neither a strict, 'cry-it-out' method (where it's suggested you just shut the door and leave the baby to it) nor a full 'contact to sleep' approach (where you co-sleep then gradually try to remove your physical presence), but a happy medium between the two. It also involves implementing some boundaries around bedtime and encouraging your child to go to sleep independently, while giving frequent 'reassurances' if they become upset and protest at the changes. It is not a long and drawn-out process, such as the gradual-retreat method, and should only take a few days and nights (depending on the child's age) to achieve a full night's sleep with the minimum of upset along the way. It's no surprise that many parents claim: 'It was the best thing we ever did!'

A PARENT'S STORY

'Although I desperately wanted the situation to change and get better, I was still really anxious about "sleep-training" as I thought the phrase sounded a little harsh, but Alison's technique is wonderful. Babies are constantly reassured, which made me feel able to see it through. My boys responded so well and were not distressed at all. It was truly remarkable to witness.'

E. W.

Based on some in-depth research of the available science, along with my own expertise and experience, I have compiled the following list of myths built up around the term 'sleep-training'; hopefully my responses will quickly dispel them and allay any worries, fears and anxieties you may have.

Myth 1 *If I let my child cry, they will hate me.*

Fact Multiple studies show that there are no negative effects on the parent–child bond from sleep-training. In fact, some studies actually show an improvement in security between parent and child following sleep-training.

Alison says 'Over the past twenty years, thousands of parents have successfully followed my reassurance sleep-training technique without negative consequences.'

Myth 2 *If I sleep-train my child, I can't hold her at night and sing to her any more.*

Fact Sleep-training does not mean giving up the activities you love to do with your child – you can continue to do them as part of the night-time routine. With sleep-training you simply avoid these activities just at the time of transition from wake to sleep.

Alison says 'Establishing a positive bedtime routine before sleep is helpful to promote positive sleep associations and can include story-time, songs, hugs, kisses and cuddles.'

Myth 3 *Sleep-training means I can't share a room with my child.*

Fact It is completely fine to sleep in the same room as the child during sleep-training, but it can make the process more difficult to see through.

Alison says 'I've helped parents who have no option but to room-share with their children, but by implementing clear boundaries you can still achieve a full night's sleep for all.'

Myth 4 Sleep-training is for the benefit of the parents, not the child.

Fact Although adults do tend to sleep better once their child is sleeping, it is not implemented for the benefit of the parents. Proper sleep is necessary for the child's healthy development in all areas.

Alison says 'All my advice on everything sleep-related is child-focused and follows their natural needs, biological clock and sleep rhythms.'

Myth 5 There are long-term risks to sleep-training.

Fact Scientific research has found there are no reported long-term risks from sleep-training. Rather, there are multiple studies showing both short- and long-term improvements in sleep-quality for children and in parents' mental well-being.

Alison says 'Sadly, I have witnessed many instances of babies and toddlers who did gain a phobia of bedtime and sleep due to previous sleep-training attempts. However, this was nearly always because the baby or child actually had underlying and undiagnosed digestive discomfort related to acid-reflux and/or dietary intolerances, which prevented them being able to sleep comfortably and which, in turn, made them fearful of going to bed and sleeping.'

Myth 6 After I sleep-train, my child will sleep through the night.

Fact No human being actually stays fast asleep the entire night. We are roused multiple times every hour, when we might fidget or turn over. Even after sleep-training, children will wake up throughout the night and may roll over, move briefly or make noises, but the key is that, after sleep-training, they will be able to put themselves back to sleep after these natural wakings.

Alison says 'The key to children sleeping through is for them to feel safe and secure, and to be able to self-soothe and go back to sleep without needing help when they naturally wake at various times throughout the night.'

Myth 7 I don't need to sleep-train because my child will grow out of it within a few months.

Fact While it is true that most children will eventually stop needing help to fall asleep, the timing varies greatly. It is not unusual for five- and six-year-olds to still wake up multiple times and want to be fed or rocked to get back to sleep, and there are even teenagers who still insist on sleeping next to their parents to fall asleep. The child may outgrow it eventually, but in the worst-case scenario it might only be when they leave home.

Alison says 'So many parents simply hang on for the age at which their child is supposed to miraculously "outgrow" their night-time wakings and suddenly produce a full 12-hour-night's sleep, but my advice is to find out *why* your child is resisting sleep, as once you discover the reason you can more quickly find the solution.'

Myth 8 Sleep-training prescribes a set, optimum number of minutes between visits to a toddler's room.

Fact There isn't any scientific data showing whether going in after three minutes or ten minutes will give a quicker or more effective result than checking more or less often. The amount of time you leave depends much more on what you, as the parent, feel comfortable with. I'm sure if the child is your first-born you will be checking much more frequently than with your second or third child, whom you will be more comfortable to leave for longer.

Alison says 'In my first book I included a "crying scale" that I devised to help parents interpret their baby's cry so they could work out how and when to respond throughout the sleep-training process. This scale is still useful for those sleep-training older children, so I have included it in this book, too (see p. 170).

Myth 9 Sleep-training involves leaving a child to cry themselves to sleep.

Fact For those who are adamantly opposed to letting a child cry but are frustrated by the lack of consistent sleep, there are other sleep-training techniques that don't involve leaving an infant to cry. It's up to you to research which method is going to suit you best.

Alison says 'My technique is not just about closing the door and letting a child cry, but there are sometimes tears. You cannot explain to a toddler why you are changing things and putting them into their own bed, removing their middle-of-the-night milk feed or their beloved dummy, and the change is likely to cause a little upset for the first night or two. Most parents report back after implementing my method to say it was nowhere near as awful as they had previously expected! All the evidence suggests that lack of sleep has a negative impact on a child's health, mood and development in the long term, and no study states that sleep-training has any harmful effects.'

Let us also remember that, whatever form of parenting we choose – whether we co-sleep or not, sleep-train or not, and, if we do sleep-train, whatever method we might choose to do this – no one has the right to judge us, criticize or comment on our choices or actions. Your parenting style is entirely your decision and one that you will have made with the best intentions, doing only what feels right for you and your family. So, try not to worry that others won't approve of your choices; it's not up to them, it's up to you and you alone. Meanwhile, treat others the way you wish to be treated: be kind, be considerate, be supportive. And, most of all, be happy in yourself and with the decisions you make throughout your parenting journey.

HOW MUCH SLEEP? SCHEDULES AND ROUTINES

The amount of sleep we each require varies, particularly when we become adults, but, according to the Mental Health Foundation, research makes it clear that getting enough sleep is essential at all ages. Sleep powers the mind and restores the body, fortifying virtually every system within it. But how much sleep do we really need in order to get these benefits? It is estimated that healthy adults need 7–9 hours of sleep per night (7–8 hours for those over 65), but to ensure healthy growth and development, babies, young children and teenagers need considerably more.

The following table sets out the total expected daily sleep requirements for older babies, toddlers and young children. Based on the average amount for each age group, it also shows how many daytime naps are needed to promote good night-time sleep.

Age	Total hours	Night-time sleep	Daytime naps
6–12 months	15–17	12	2 naps
12–18 months	14–15	12	1–2 naps
18–24 months	13–15	12–13	1 nap
2–3.5 years	12–14	12–13	1 nap
3.5–5 years	11–13	11–13	0 naps

Of course, there will be individual variation in how your toddler's sleep patterns develop – for example, whether at twelve months they have decided to have just one, longer nap during the day or to continue to enjoy two naps; either is more than acceptable. The key to daytime sleep, and whether they are getting the right amount and at the right time, needs to be guided by what's happening at night.

For example, if your twelve-month-old is waking at 5am after barely sleeping 10 hours at night, but is then needing two 3-hour naps during the day, logic tells us his patterns are slightly off-kilter. In some ways this scenario isn't disastrous but it will start to interfere with the natural activities of the day. Starting your day so early is tiring, and trying to incorporate these two long naps for your toddler along with managing nursery runs for an older child or attending social toddler classes, for example, will likely prove quite challenging.

In my first book, *The Sensational Baby Sleep Plan*, I talk about following a natural, 12-hour day/night split and using the timings of 7am–7pm. Many parents opt to do either a 6am–6pm or an 8am–8pm schedule, which is absolutely fine, but do look at what your day will look like once you return to work or your older child starts nursery or school. Starting your day at 8am may well be too late to get everyone fully organized and ready to leave the house by 8.45am, for example, and although you can adapt your little one's body clock further down the line, it's better to start off with the timings that, for the most part, your household needs to follow for the longer term.

Of course, while having a daily routine is important, it need only be a guide to follow, as opposed to a strictly timed and regimented plan. After all, each day is never exactly the same as the one before, and indeed, who knows what tomorrow will bring?

This table gives a suggested daily schedule based on the average expectation of natural sleep and mealtime requirements at different ages.

	6–12 months	12–18 months	18–24 months	2–3.5 years	3.5–5 years
7am	Milk	Milk/ Water	Water	Water	Water
8am			Breakfast	Breakfast	Breakfast
8.30am	Breakfast	Breakfast			
9am	Nap 1–2 hours	Nap 30–60 minutes			
10am		Snack/ Drink	Snack/ Drink	Snack/ Drink	Snack/ Drink
11am	Milk stopping as solids take over				
12 noon	Lunch	Lunch	Lunch	Lunch	Lunch

	6–12 months	12–18 months	18–24 months	2–3.5 years	3.5–5 years
12.30pm		Nap 2–3 hours . . .	Nap 2 hours	Nap 1–2 hours	
1pm	Nap 1.5–2 hours	. . . Or nap here			
2.30/3pm	Milk	Milk/ Snack	Snack/ Drink	Snack/ Drink	Snack/ Drink
4.30/5.30pm	Dinner	Dinner	Dinner	Dinner	Dinner
6pm	Bath	Bath	Bath	Bath	Bath
6.30pm	Milk	Milk	Milk	Milk/ Water	Milk/ Water
6.45pm	Story and bed				
7pm		Story and bed	Story and bed	Story and bed	
7.30pm					Story and bed

As you can see, there is room for variation. Some toddlers may have given up all milk feeds by the time they are twelve or eighteen months old, while others might continue to have milk at bedtime until they are three. Equally, naps will vary from child to child, but essentially one would expect them still to have one daytime nap until around three years of age.

Of course, having written this book during the Covid-19 pandemic, I am fully aware of how different life has been, and may continue to be for some time to come. There have been huge changes to daily life, with children not going to school, parents on furlough and not going out to work, others working from home and sadly many people being very unwell while still trying to cope and care for their children, often with little or no help. In such circumstances sometimes routines, schedules and boundaries may need to be relaxed while you just try to cope from one day to the next, or need to recover from being unwell.

A PARENT'S STORY

'The journey back from having Covid hasn't been as smooth as I'd naively anticipated it would be. I felt tiredness before it – as a parent, I'm accustomed to feeling tired all the time – but this particular type of exhaustion has been something else. It comes in waves and it just cripples you. I'm a busy bee by nature, so I'm finding this really frustrating. I've literally been doing whatever it takes to get through the day right now, with my priority being to rest. The TV has become a reliable childminder and it's been "yes" to whatever the kids want. Every routine has been out the window, with the baby sleeping next to me as I simply have no energy to battle it out to put her in the cot. I've thrown away all guilt, as it wasn't serving anyone, and accepted that right now this is my reality and prioritizing rest is what will get me better.'

P. K.

The above quote was Instagrammed by the GP Dr Punam Krishan. Punam goes on to admit that when she goes back to work, some kind of normal, daily routine will need to be re-established for the children. Such returns to normality after a period of interruption to daily life can often take a few days, with various levels of protest from the little ones as you try to get them back on track, but with a sense of calm, plenty of patience, much resolve and clear instruction, routines and boundaries for your little ones can certainly be reset.

DAYTIME NAPS AND QUIET-TIME

So many parents feel a lot of stress about implementing and achieving daytime naps with their little ones. In the early months, naps will rarely fall into a routine until a full night's sleep is properly established. Many will follow advice to wake their baby after a 45-minute morning nap, enforce a 2-hour sleep after lunch and/or not let their baby nap again after 4pm, but often with little success as these strict timings, and the restriction of sleep for the first daytime nap and later in the day, are not aligned with the baby's natural sleep patterns.

My advice is somewhat different from most, because I suggest you implement a more flexible nap structure that better follows your baby's natural sleep patterns. During the first 8–10 months, the easiest daytime nap to establish is the first one of the day. It's also the most rejuvenating and the best-quality daytime sleep your little one will have, even after a full, 12-hour sleep at night. This often means that the after-lunch daytime nap that most parents try to achieve may not be quite so successful and may be frustratingly variable in its length. However, as your baby heads to twelve months old the need for two daytime naps will lessen and by eighteen months you can expect your little one to be having only the one nap, after lunch, which stays in place for another year or so.

Let's look at the expected nap structure in more detail.

At 6 months Around this time, if you've followed *The Sensational Baby Sleep Plan*, I would expect your baby to be ready to drop the late-afternoon nap, which will have been established from the very early weeks, and now require just two naps each day, one in the morning and one after lunch. To cope with the longer afternoon, from wake-up after the second nap through to bedtime, you can push back the timings of the naps so that the first is at around 9/9.30am instead of 8.30am, and then the second nap starts at around 1/1.30pm instead of 12.30.

Approaching 12 months Some babies seem to need to drop the morning nap around this time, though some do it sooner, or later, than others – the earliest I have seen was at ten months and there are some who keep two naps until they're almost two!

2–3.5 years Once your little one is down to just the one, after-lunch nap as they head towards three years old, they may then drop the nap completely. The earliest I would expect a toddler to be able to do without the nap is around two and a half years, whereas some will keep their beloved nap until around three and a half.

Working out when and how to drop from two naps to one, and then deciding that your child doesn't need the daytime nap at all, can be quite tricky and there is no exact age to be guided by. However, if your older baby is sleeping from 9–10.30am in the morning and suddenly starts to not sleep easily for his second nap, or is sleeping then for only 30–45 minutes, it's a sure sign that you need to limit the morning nap to promote a better after-lunch sleep. Start by waking your baby 15 minutes before his usual wake-up time at the first nap and see what, if any, effect that has on the second nap. If there's not much change, limit the first nap to just 1 hour or even 45 minutes, which should then help him to sleep better for his second nap.

Once this transition has taken place, it is likely that after a few weeks he will no longer need the first morning nap at all, and he will settle down to the one-nap strategy. Instead of putting your little one down at the usual time of 9–9.30am, keep him up for as long as you can before you feel he needs to sleep. This transitional phase can take a week or so and lunch can become somewhat interrupted, so you may need to alter the timings of his meal for a few days. For example, if your little one can only manage to get to 11am before he really needs to sleep, give him a good mid-morning snack beforehand then another robust snack, or a late lunch, once he wakes from his nap. As he may have gone to sleep at 11am and woken at, say, 1.30pm, the slightly longer afternoon may also be a tad challenging as he gets increasingly tired and grumpy heading towards 6pm. You can always do an earlier bath and bedtime for a few days to compensate, but hopefully it will all fall into place within a week or so and he will easily be able to wait for lunch at 12pm then go down for his nap at around 12.30, then you can re-establish the usual bedtime.

Somewhere between two and a half and three and half years of age, your toddler will reach the point when he doesn't need a daytime nap at all, and although you may be dreading this and miss having that glorious hour or so to yourself, I'm afraid it will happen at some point! The usual indications that the nap needs to be shortened or stopped are when your toddler:

- suddenly protests at being put to bed for the nap

- happily goes to bed but just doesn't sleep, or wakes after a short time

- doesn't want to go to bed at night

- stays awake until later in the evening and seems unable to fall asleep at the usual night-time bedtime

- randomly wakes in the night

- wakes too early in the morning and is unable to sleep through to the usual 7am

- sleeps erratically for the daytime nap, sleeping one day but not the next, then might not sleep at all until nodding off in the car or pushchair later in the day – or even over their meal at 5pm!

Once it becomes evident that your toddler is no longer going to sleep for his daytime nap, I advise trying to keep some 'quiet-time' in place as it can be hugely beneficial, relaxing him and allowing his system to rest a little and recharge, ready to face the rest of the day.

However, trying to establish quiet-time can, in reality, prove to be quite challenging so here are some tips for implementing it:

- **Decide the duration and stick to it.** Decide how long you want the 'quiet-time' to last and make it the same every day. You could choose to make it a minimum of 30 minutes, but I feel at least 60 minutes is more beneficial, perhaps even 90 minutes for the first few months. As your child gets older, the need for quiet-time will lessen and you can reduce the length of the session until you no longer feel it's beneficial.

- **Choose a setting.** You might decide that they need to stay in their cot for quiet-time, which is easier to implement than if you've already moved them into a bed. If that's the case, you may decide that they can move around their bedroom during the session as long as they don't come out. Or you may prefer to let them have quiet-time on a sofa or quiet area of the lounge or playroom, but this can be trickier to implement because they will naturally try to engage with you or others in the household, making quiet-time rather less quiet!

- **Provide things for them to do.** Quiet-time will only be successful if you provide something to occupy your toddler; it's unrealistic to expect a two- or three-year-old just to sit on their own, either on their bed or on the sofa, with nothing to entertain them. Find books, jigsaws, shape-sorters or toys, for example, and make sure there's nothing they can damage, rip, tear or harm themselves with.

- **Avoid giving screens.** This may be the most tempting option for getting your toddler to settle for quiet-time, and while it is not the worst scenario in the world, it really is better to use another form of entertainment, even just audiobooks to listen to.

- **Use a clock or timer.** Use a clock or timer to show your toddler that it's still quiet-time. Explain that when the clock says 14:30 or the big hand reaches the two, for example, quiet-time will end. It may take a few days for them to fully understand the concept, and if you feel that they may not understand the numbers showing on a clock you could instead set an alarm to signal the end of quiet-time.

- **Supervise them via video monitor.** With modern technology, it's easy to keep a watchful eye on your little one during quiet-time through a remote video monitor or 'nanny cam', allowing you to check that they are staying safe and behaving!

- **Be consistent, every day.** If your child decides to resist quiet-time and keeps coming out of the bedroom or calling out, you will need to be resilient, putting them back in their room and refraining from engaging in conversation or responding to any unnecessary demands each and every day. In fact, this technique is very similar to that described in the next chapter for implementing sleep-training for a toddler.

THE FORBIDDEN SLEEP ZONE

Many children experience a 'second wind' an hour or so before their natural bedtime. This used to be attributed to an energy boost from food ingested at dinner time, but the latest, fascinating research into sleep has shown it to be caused by a naturally occurring 'forbidden sleep zone', a period of time where a natural wakefulness occurs shortly before the onset of nocturnal sleep.

One would think that it would be increasingly easy to fall

asleep as the day wears on, but this is not the case. While there are energy dips that happen earlier in the day – and these are particularly pronounced in babies and children, which is why they need daytime naps – as adults we can be as alert for the 2–3 hours before our usual bedtime as when we woke in the morning. This is because, during this period, the body increases its production of the thyroid-stimulating hormone thyrotropin. Some research suggests this has an evolutionary function: as night fell, this hormonal surge created an enhanced awareness within the body that allowed for a period of safety preparation – finding a place to sleep safe from predators or the elements – before settling down to sleep for the night.

Understanding this wakeful period leading up to your toddler's bedtime, and ensuring there is some energetic activity after dinner, is helpful for promoting a better night's sleep for your child. The temptation after dinner can be to sit your toddler in front of the television to give you time to clear away after the meal, but this will not be wholly conducive to an easy bedtime and a settled night's sleep, and we now know there are two reasons for this.

- As previously mentioned in Chapters 1 and 2, screen time before bed can prevent the onset of melatonin production in the body, which is a necessity for sleep.

- While watching a screen can easily distract your child from the natural need for activity after dinner time, ignoring this 'forbidden sleep zone' will prevent the natural hormonal change necessary for healthy sleep.

So, before embarking on the quieter, wind-down period of bathtime and stories, engage your toddler in some fun, energetic play – a game of hide and seek, some running races up and down the hall or in the garden, circuits around the kitchen on their trikes or bikes, a game of catch or piggy-in-the-middle with a ball, or even just some singing and dancing.

There are actually many other advantages for your child (and some for you) of such play before bedtime. It can:

- induce a feel-good factor

- use up any unspent energy before bed

- further build their connection with you, by sharing enjoyment

- assist in the release of pent-up feelings and emotions from the day

- be fun and relaxing, leaving a happy feeling in you both as bathtime approaches

- provide a working parent, particularly one away from the home all day, a great time to reconnect with your child

- help you both to forget earlier tantrums or conflict that happened during the day

- make bedtime feel more acceptable for your child after this happy, fun and positively engaging period of play

Try to build into your daily routine at least 20–30 minutes after dinner to have fun, play and burn off the energy that has naturally built up during this 'forbidden sleep zone', and end it with an active 'tidy-up' time. I always feel it is important to encourage children to take responsibility for their belongings, and having a fun tidy-up time at the end of each day – perhaps with a 'race' to see how quickly it can be done – helps your child learn to take care of their toys, games and books.

SLEEP REGRESSIONS: ARE THEY REAL?

Contrary to most other opinions, I do not believe that 'sleep regressions' are an actual *thing*. Sure, babies, toddlers and children can all experience disruptions to sleep – even those that have slept through from an early age and have been brilliant sleepers may experience periods of time when their sleep becomes erratic. But to suggest, as many do, that all babies and children will, at the same specific age, experience a developmental leap that will lead to a regression in their sleep habits seems, to me, extremely unlikely.

While infants' brains do seem to go through periods of explosive growth during their first two years, no verifiable studies solidly identified which specific changes happen in which specific weeks. So, while experts and parents agree that sleep patterns can vary wildly throughout a child's first two years, there is no rigorous data that supports the notion that nap- and night-time sleep changes happen at predetermined times or are linked to specific developmental milestones.

ALISON SAYS . . .

'I hear from so many parents who, even when their baby is sleeping beautifully and as expected, both at night and for day naps, are constantly on edge, waiting for it all to regress due to a supposed developmental leap and sleep regression that they've been told is fast-approaching!'

NIGHT-TIME WAKINGS

There are many reasons why your toddler might have suddenly started to wake during the night, is not settling for naps or bedtime or is perhaps resisting any sleep, and it's important to work out why this has happened, rather than excuse it as a 'developmental leap' or some expected 'sleep regression'.

Typical factors that may affect or disturb your toddler's sleep include:

- onset of teething

- being unwell or brewing an illness

- not wanting to sleep in a cot

- moving into a big bed

- daytime naps that have been longer than necessary, or could be dropped

- starting nursery

- the arrival of a sibling

- an extended disruption to routine, such as Christmas festivities

- the excitement of an approaching birthday

- moving home

- being on holiday/travelling

- a change in family life or the home situation

- a life trauma, such as a family member passing away

- a dietary change

- having watched a TV programme that caused some upset in your child

- experiencing an unpleasant interaction with another child

- separation anxiety

- too much screen time

- feelings of anxiety or stress

- acid-reflux or digestive discomfort due to food allergies or intolerances

Often it is fairly easy to understand why your toddler is feeling unsettled – due, perhaps, to starting nursery or moving home – but at other times it may be more difficult to work out the reason. For example, chicken pox has an incubation period during which your little one may feel quite unwell and not sleep easily, but with no obvious symptoms until the spots erupt two to three weeks later. Similarly, perhaps there is a disruption to sleep with no obvious explanation for a few days, but then your toddler suddenly sprouts a new molar.

With nearly every phase of disrupted sleep there will be an underlying cause, and you will often need to put on your 'detective hat' to work out what it is. Take a step back and look at any changes you may have made during the last few weeks, whether to diet, routine or daily life, and try to understand what your toddler is really trying to tell you. Once you can determine the underlying cause, it is obviously then easier to address and resolve the situation, and, following the techniques detailed in the next chapter, continuous sleep should quickly be restored.

Depending on the underlying issue, you may need to adapt the techniques before attempting to implement them but, quite often, once the root cause of the sleep problem has been addressed, very little actual sleep-training is needed.

The following are two common causes of night-time wakings that can be resolved without sleep-training.

Transition to cow's milk

Following the current NHS guidelines, many parents switch their baby's milk to full-fat, ordinary cow's milk at twelve months. However, this can often cause a disruption to sleep because cow's milk is so difficult for babies to digest and creates some degree of tummy discomfort. It doesn't necessarily mean that your baby is allergic or fully intolerant to cow's milk, but that they are simply unable to cope with the increased volume of the full-fat cow's milk at bedtime. If you make this switch from ordinary formula or breast milk and over the following few weeks your little one starts waking during the night, try switching back or using a plant-based milk instead, to see if it resolves the night-time wakings. As soon as your child's tummy is having its normal milk again, he should hopefully revert back to comfortable sleep. You could then try to reintroduce cow's milk a few months later by adding it to solid food rather than giving an actual drink of milk.

Teething

Teething can often cause a disturbance to sleep, and sadly there's little you can really do except give some pain relief where appropriate or use teething gels, or give your little one a teether to chomp on, perhaps with some teething gel on it, and leave it with them in their cot or bed at night. During periods of teething, try to resettle your little one as best you can and once the offending tooth has appeared, all should quite easily return to normal, with sound sleep restored.

Holding back

All too often, you can be caught off-guard by your toddler suddenly waking up in the middle of the night, completely out of the blue. On hearing her cry, your immediate reaction will be to rush into her bedroom to see what's happened. However, if at all possible, try to refrain from dashing straight into the room, but just wait a few minutes, watch on the video camera if you have one and try to work out what could have disturbed her.

Obviously, if you feel you need to check on your child then do so, but it is much more preferable to compose yourself a little first and try to adopt a calm aura before going in. Your child may already be upset because of a bad dream or a loud noise that startled and woke her, and if you are then obviously flustered and anxious too, this can add to your little one's feelings of unease and actually make matters worse. It is very easy to overreact, panic and try to do too much, too soon, to calm and soothe your child, but if you had perhaps waited for a few minutes before rushing in, she might have resettled herself quite easily and not actually needed any intervention from you.

ALISON SAYS . . .

'While it's fantastic if you have a child who is a brilliant sleeper and never wakes at night, always be prepared for the unexpected! If there ever is a night-time waking, try not to rush into the room in a panic, but rather wait a minute or two and try to assess the situation, then work out what may be the cause. Obviously you will need to tend to your child as appropriate to the circumstances, but try and manage the situation as calmly as possible.'

BEDTIME FEARS, NIGHTMARES AND NIGHT TERRORS

Bedtime fears, nightmares and night terrors are three different problems that toddlers and young children may experience. From around the age of two, children, like adults, dream during REM sleep, but in some cases these dreams can to turn into nightmares, with a few children developing night terrors. As children get older, fears around going to bed can also sometimes start to build.

Babies younger than two also have an REM sleep cycle but some neuroscientists believe that it is designed simply to develop the neural pathways and connections needed. If this is the case and young babies don't dream, it would be safe to say that they do not have nightmares either.

For a number of reasons, it's tricky to know what young children dream about. It's a challenge even for researchers who study childhood dreams, because:

- The child might leave out key details.

- They might be shy and not want to talk about the experience at all.

- They might not have the words to fully explain their dream.

- They may exaggerate what they believe they remember.

- They may tell you a story unrelated to their dream.

Psychologist David Foulkes, who studies children's sleep and is the author of *Children's Dreaming and the Development of Consciousness*, says that 'basically little children have little dreams and exactly what they see while dreaming depends on their age. As children develop and grow, their dreams do too.'

What we do know is that all dreams have one important thing in common: they are very accurate at relating emotional issues within our lives. Our dreams especially reflect our fears, and tend to be based on visual experiences. In addition, a person's individual lived experience will create the background and detail to the dream, so it's believed that because young children have not had much 'life experience' their dreams are fairly basic. Toddler dreams feature animals and familiar sights such as children playing or people eating. According to David Foulkes, 'Children dream life – the life they live and events that occur in it are recreated within their dreams.'

For a child, a nightmare will usually begin as a normal dream, but as it progresses the images and feelings induced by it turn into something frightening. For example, your child may dream that he was happily playing in the park (which relates to something that has actually happened during the day), when it suddenly starts to get dark or he can't see you and feels totally alone, then others in the park might turn into scary people or even monsters.

Understanding the fact that 'children dream life' makes it somewhat obvious that if children have frightening experiences, witness arguments, live with anger, are neglected, bullied or abused, then their dreams are going to reflect this and they may experience nightmares.

Thankfully, the majority of children do not experience these negative extremes, but many of them living in warm and loving environments can still experience nightmares. This is because they reflect emotional conflicts that arise in the child's waking life, many of which are just the usual struggles children face throughout their development. It is for this reason that most children will have nightmares at one time or another, whether they experience trauma within their life or not.

The specific content or the story created within your toddler's dream depends on a few factors:

- his age

- his stage of physical development

- his stage of emotional development

- any stressful situations he may have had to cope with

- any emotional conflicts he may have experienced during the day

- any scary or threatening events he may have experienced recently

It is quite normal for young children to develop fears around going to bed, and most do so at some point during childhood. There are so many issues within normal daily life that your toddler has to learn to understand and manage (many being the same that cause night-time wakings, as listed on p. 91), and the anxieties that can lead to the development of nightmares can also induce fears around bedtime. Your toddler may protest during the evening routine, not want to go to bed or not fall asleep easily and become quite upset.

If a sudden fear of the dark or not wanting to fall asleep alone is causing bedtime troubles, then you might decide to adopt some of the following tactics:

- Gently encourage your child to talk about what might be upsetting her, but don't force the issue if she doesn't want to discuss it.

- If she describes a fear of monsters, for example, it's important that you don't support these fears. By 'cleaning the room of monsters' or doing an 'under-bed monster sweep' you are inadvertently agreeing that the monsters exist, which fuels her belief that they are real.

It is far better to explain during the day that monsters are not real and just made up for books and cartoons.

- You could introduce a comforter such as a weighted blanket, a cuddle-cushion or a cuddly toy. There's more information on these ideas in the night-time disturbances section (on p. 138).

- A low, glowing night-light placed in the room can help and is preferable to leaving the bedroom door open for a light source.

- Avoid letting her watch any 'scary' television shows or videos or showing her any picture books that could increase bedtime fears.

Night terrors are very different from nightmares. A child having a night terror may scream, shout, thrash around, seem to be completely panicked or even jump out of bed and not recognize you if you try to comfort them. The child's eyes will often be open but they're not fully awake during these episodes and will likely have no memory of it in the morning. The episodes usually happen in the early part of the night, continue for a few minutes (sometimes as long as 15) and can occur more than once a night. While nightmares occur in REM sleep, night terrors occur when a child wakes abruptly from deep, non-REM sleep, with possible triggers being a sudden noise, general overexcitement or anxiety, or just a full bladder. They can also be induced by a high fever or certain types of medication.

The best thing to do if your child is having an episode of night terrors is to stay calm and wait patiently until they calm down; try not to intervene, interact with or wake them unless they are not safe – they may become even more agitated if you try to comfort them. Although they can be frightening to witness, night terrors don't really harm your child and it's likely that your child won't remember the episode the next morning.

Thankfully, true night terrors do not occur with any frequency and often stop as quickly as they start, but if they continue or intensify then it would be important to try and find out why they are happening, what could be triggering them and if there's anything you can do to prevent them.

You may need to seek help from a GP to rule out any possibility that they may be caused by a medical condition, for example:

- enlarged tonsils causing restricted breathing
- inflamed adenoids leading to sleep apnoea
- build-up of fluid or wax in the ear, or a possible ear infection
- acid-reflux causing internal pain and discomfort (NB: the above three conditions are usually linked to, and caused by, acid damage from some degree of reflux.)
- a urine or kidney infection
- a dietary allergy or intolerance

It is also important to look at other aspects of your child's daily life and find out whether there is something causing distress, upset or anxiety – at nursery or school, for example – that could also be the underlying reason for the night terrors happening.

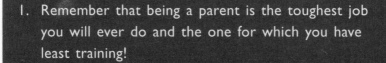

☆ ALISON'S GOLDEN RULES ☆

1. Remember that being a parent is the toughest job you will ever do and the one for which you have least training!

2. Try not to impose your own anxieties around sleep on your child, and know that most sleep problems are not hereditary.

3. Remember that sleep deprivation is incredibly damaging both to your own health and that of your child, whereas short-term sleep-training is proven to have no negative long-term effects.

4. Always try to find out *why* your child is not sleeping. Put on your 'detective hat' and investigate the possible causes.

5. Try to stay calm and be patient if your child is resisting sleep – the more anxious you become, the more upset your child will be too.

6. Believe that your toddler is capable of sleeping well; you just need to give the right cues and environment.

7. If your child is sleeping well, then enjoy the peace and don't stress about supposed looming sleep regressions – they don't exist!

8. Create a fun playtime between dinner and bathtime, and end the session with an active 'tidy-up' time where you put away all the toys and books enjoyed during the day.

9. Keep bedtime fairly simple – bath, milk, teeth-brushing, stories, kisses and cuddles and then 'Goodnight' – and make it the same time each night.

10. Try not to panic or overreact to any night-time wakings. Take a deep breath, lower your shoulders and adopt a calm aura before trying to manage the situation.

CHAPTER 4

Before You Start Sleep-training

I hope that the first three chapters will have given you enough information to understand the science behind sleep and the natural sleep requirements for your toddler. They should also have provided a basis for creating boundaries, setting a daytime routine and better managing certain aspects of your child's behaviour, all of which will help to promote positive sleep associations for the longer term.

This chapter and the following one will give you full practical guidance on how to establish a full night's sleep, resolve sleep issues with your little one and restore peaceful evenings to your household. You will discover how to implement my reassurance sleep-training, adapt it according to the age of your child and ensure it is appropriate for your individual situation and circumstances.

WHY SLEEP PROBLEMS HAPPEN

There are many different reasons why your toddler may not have learned to sleep through the night, or, having done so for some time, has now started to resist bedtime and wake during the night:

- You may not have followed my plan or, indeed, implemented any kind of routine, and consequently your little one has not yet learned to sleep through the night.

- Perhaps your toddler has never been a good daytime sleeper and, as a result, doesn't sleep well at night either, due to being so overtired.

- You may have decided to co-sleep in the earlier months, and though you want to change things now, your little one cannot seem to sleep alone.

- You may have been offering the 'dream feed' (a feed given just before you go to bed) or are continuing to give night feeds, which your little one now relies upon and is reluctant to give up.

- Your child may be reliant on a dummy, which actively encourages her to wake up when she loses it and then requires your intervention to help find it.

- Perhaps your little one has become attached to a comforter (a cuddly toy or 'blankie', for example) that has somehow got lost in the daytime and he now won't settle without it.

- Perhaps your toddler struggled with acid-reflux as a baby and still has unmanaged symptoms, which are interfering with their night-time sleep – because, contrary to popular belief, many babies do not just 'outgrow' it.

- Your child may have food allergies or intolerances that cause digestive discomfort and prevent him from sleeping easily at night.

- Perhaps your toddler is teething, unwell or has some other medical problem that interferes with sleep.

- The arrival of another baby can easily unsettle your toddler and may cause him to display some negative reactions, including waking at night.

- Any change in your toddler's usual environment, such as a new home or a trip away for the weekend, can cause him to be less settled at night.

- Being on holiday, staying with friends or family, travelling abroad and encountering different time-zones may cause your toddler to fall out of their routine, making them more unable to sleep as soundly as when at home.

- The hour-change that takes place in the UK every March and October can cause disruption to your toddler's sleep.

- Your child may have started nursery or school or changed classroom, leaving her feeling somewhat apprehensive and perhaps experiencing a degree of separation anxiety, which means she is less happy to sleep at night.

- A change in your family dynamics, when you are dealing with a bereavement, a family split or any other stressful situation life throws at you, may result in your toddler picking up on a tense atmosphere and feeling more unsettled, especially at night.

Whatever the cause of your toddler's sleep problems, it can seem like a hopeless situation when, no matter what you have tried, nothing seems to help. All too often I hear parents declare that they have the child who doesn't need sleep, or they are convinced that their child is 'different' in some way and there is no sleep solution for them. In fact, nearly every parent who has asked for my help has felt that way and has been sure that their toddler will be the only one who will not respond to my reassurance sleep-training technique! Happily they have all been wrong and, although some children along the way have proved to be quite 'challenging', many more have responded with ease.

Being consistent

With such a wide variety of advice available, many parents will have tried a multitude of methods over a number of days, nights, weeks or even months to try to get their toddler to go to sleep easily and sleep through the night. When things aren't resolved as the weeks roll on, and sleep becomes even more elusive, parents become increasingly desperate, constantly trying more 'sleep remedies' in the hope that one may resolve the situation, usually to no avail. A big problem with repeated experimentation is the lack of consistency that builds as parents set out with determination each night to try a new method of sleep-training and stick to it, but come the early hours they 'give in' and revert to giving the begged-for milk, for example, or taking the child into their bed.

Unfortunately, the more things you try, the more your toddler will become confused and be unable to understand what you expect of them each night, as the rules around sleep change too frequently. Perhaps you'll recognize some of the following scenarios:

- You lie next to your toddler as she goes to sleep, but other nights try to make her go to sleep alone.

- You give her milk every time she wakes, but some nights substitute it with water or try to make her go back to sleep without anything to drink at all.

- You allow your toddler into your bed when she wakes in the early hours, but on other occasions make her stay in her own room.

- On some nights you try to bribe her with a treat in the morning if she sleeps through – and even if she didn't sleep you still give the treat anyway!

- Sitting in her room or standing by the door while she goes to sleep might have worked, but then you have to resume the position every time she wakes, so some nights you try to stay away from her room; others you just give in and sleep on her floor.

- Some nights you might give in and read the twenty stories she demanded before going to sleep, but on others you try to read her only one.

- Sometimes you might try a light show, a night-light or playing soothing music – and when it doesn't seem to work, stop using them.

- You might leave the door open as per her demands, but then threaten to close it if she doesn't go to sleep – sometimes closing it, sometimes not.

- In desperation, you might resort to putting a lock on her bedroom door or putting up a stair-gate to stop her coming out of the room, but then feel guilty about doing so and take them away. (NB: In my opinion it's absolutely fine to put up a stair-gate or lock the door to prevent your child from opening the door, especially if there's a safety issue such as a steep staircase that your little one could fall down.)

- Perhaps you implemented a reward chart but still give a star or sticker in the morning, even if she got up in the night, or just stopped using it when the novelty wore off.

- Some nights you might lose your patience and end up shouting at her, whereas others you try to soothe, comfort and talk to her in the hope she will sleep.

These are just a few situations I've witnessed or heard about, and if they sound familiar it's no wonder your toddler hasn't a clue how to behave at night! However, by using my reassurance sleep-training technique, you will be able to eradicate all this confusion and reinforce one simple message: it's sleepy-time!

A PARENT'S STORY

'Owing to my wife being very unwell with Covid-19, I got into bad habits with our toddler and reverted to letting him fall asleep on me in his room at bedtime so we wouldn't disturb my wife in the next room. Looking after my sick wife and trying to manage our toddler was really tricky and it caused me to create such strong contact-sleep associations for my son that I didn't think he would ever sleep independently again. But Alison's plan worked amazingly. It took three nights, during which our toddler cried with various levels of protest, but I can now walk out of the room after saying "goodnight" and he falls asleep in his bed, on his own and we are downstairs by 7.10pm each evening.'

D. W.

Promoting positive associations with bedtime and sleep

A major factor that can perpetuate sleep issues is the amount of focus and attention that the situation is continually given. After months of broken or little sleep, the fractious bed- and night-time antics slowly become the main topic of conversation in the household and 'the problem' is often talked about and discussed at every opportunity. It may be the first conversation with your child as you start your day, with such questions or comments as:

- 'How come you wouldn't sleep?'

- 'Why do you keep getting up?'

- 'We talk about this every day and you always promise Mummy that you will be a good girl from now on!'

- 'I don't know how I'm going to get through the day; we are all so tired.'

- 'When are you going to learn to stay in your own bed?'

- 'We will buy you a new toy when you sleep through.'

- 'Are you scared of something? Perhaps we will put a light on tonight.'

I've witnessed first-hand how sleep – or the lack of it – quickly becomes the main talking point between parents too. They will discuss each night in detail, scrutinizing their actions and questioning their approach as they search for answers.

- 'Is the room too hot? Or too cold?'

- 'Shall we get a plumber in to look at the water system? It might be the noise that's waking her up.'

- 'It's your fault – you cuddle her too much.'

- 'Maybe it's the squeaky floorboards as we go upstairs?'

- 'Why did you give in and bring her to our room?'

- 'What can we try next? Perhaps we should just let her cry it out?'

- 'Shall we go to the doctor's and see if they can help?'

Every morning, many sleep-deprived parents make statements like these and heated discussions follow as they try to make sense of their seemingly hopeless and increasingly desperate situation. Then, of course, the whole night-time scenario is re-lived and explained in detail to the friend who happens to pop round or to another family member who calls.

A PARENT'S STORY

'We hadn't slept for two-and-a-half years! Our daughter simply refused to conform to *any* method of sleep-training we tried, and much as we felt we should be able to resolve things ourselves, we couldn't. We talked about it incessantly: the night-time nightmare was all we ever discussed. So we finally cracked. I called Alison, who explained that all the sleep "problems" we had with our daughter were due to underlying acid-reflux problems and food intolerances. After addressing these issues and following Alison's brilliant advice, we now have full consistency in our approach. We implemented some very clear boundaries, have a set bedtime routine and our daughter has responded so well. She goes to bed, sleeps through the night and stays there until we get her up in the morning – it's a complete miracle! What also helped was understanding that we shouldn't discuss what happened at night with each other or family members, and certainly never in front of our daughter. It's such a relief – not only that she is sleeping, but that the drama surrounding the sleep problem has been removed for all of us.'

G. M.

As the sleep problem becomes the favoured topic of conversation within the household, it also becomes a mainstay of everyday life that children quickly accept, a normal part of their day, and although it induces stress and anxiety for all, children can find validation from it. After all, at least they are being talked about! It is a well-known fact, accepted by most parenting experts, that children crave and thrive upon all attention, whether negative or positive. When attention is meted out because of bedtime refusal or constant night-time wakings, the child can often be impelled to continue with the behaviour because they gain so much attention.

It is easy, then, for the problems surrounding sleep to become a habit, with the child unable to understand how to change things themselves. They might converse with you, saying, 'Yes, Mummy, I will sleep and be a good girl tonight,' with good intention, but they just don't have the skills in their developmental toolbox to do it.

Change has to come from the parents giving clear direction, creating boundaries and instigating a non-negotiable plan. The child will then form new habits and the problems surrounding sleep will become a thing of the past.

ALISON SAYS . . .

'Many parents wait for their child to talk before they address their sleep problems, thinking they can reason with their toddler to improve sleep habits, but sadly this is a misguided belief. Toddlers and young children are simply incapable of changing ingrained and learned behaviours by discussion alone; they need to be shown how to change things and can then follow your lead.'

An important aspect of trying to structure and establish good night-time sleep for your toddler is setting a bedtime routine – one of the fundamental parts of *The Sensational Baby Sleep Plan*. If you establish the end-of-the-day sequence of bath, milk, story and bed for a younger baby, it remains the accepted prelude to night-sleeping for years to come. If you haven't done this, it's never too late to establish a routine with an older baby or toddler; it will just take a little time, patience and perseverance! The key is not to deviate from the pattern you set and not to give in to any excessive demands. Your child will likely want one more story, cuddle, kiss, drink, etc., and it's natural for them to test the boundaries. But it's up to you to keep them in place.

Ensuring a regular daytime routine, including set times for meals, snacks, milk and water, along with a nap or quiet-time, will also be important to establish positive night-time sleep associations. Chaotic schedules are known to encourage a sense of unrest in toddlers, and can make them more susceptible to meltdowns.

Overstimulation

Toddlers also struggle with overstimulation, and although parents may want to fill their children's days with fun, exciting, high-energy outings, they often need quieter days, when they are happier to be at home with some calmer, one-to-one activities. Over-stimulating your toddler during the day will only hinder your attempts to create a calm and peaceful bedtime routine as you try to implement the new approach to sleep. Many parents whose little ones usually sleep well know that on days where there's been a change of routine – an exciting event like a birthday party, or a long and stimulating day out – that night's sleep may prove elusive. Their toddler struggles to calm down and 'switch off', having been thoroughly overexcited, which in turn causes an adrenaline rush and an increase in cortisol levels.

Of course, getting out in the fresh air, meeting with friends and other parents, and socializing your little one is hugely important for a toddler (and not least for your own sanity), but it's always best, as with most things in life, to have a balance, with plenty of peaceful days too.

There are four main reasons why toddlers can become over-stimulated:

- not enough sleep

- no proper routine

- disruption to routine

- too much activity

Typical signs that a toddler is overstimulated are when they are:

- being irrational

- forgetting manners

- becoming defiant

- crying and losing control

Here are some tips to help manage an overstimulated toddler:

- Try to remain calm yourself. Children follow our lead, and when we get upset and agitated in response to them, it promotes similar behaviour.

- Reduce the noise and activity around your child. Turn off the television or music, or remove the device.

- Try to help your child put their feelings into words. Acknowledge that they are upset or angry, and try not to tell them to 'Stop it!'

- If possible, distract your child with a calming activity. Often their curiosity will make them forget their angst, as they see you perhaps looking at one of their books or toys by yourself and making comments on the story or object in your hands.

- Get outside for a gentle stroll or head into the garden for a change of scenery and some fresh air.

If all else fails, ask a friend, a grandparent or anyone else available to come and take over while you have a couple of hours off!

UNDERSTANDING SOME COMMON SLEEP ISSUES

Sleep regressions This has become a big buzz phrase, and in my opinion the term is often used to excuse poor sleep habits. It seems that if you can explain your toddler's sleep setback as an age-determined sleep regression then the understanding is that it's not something you can control or alter! However, I believe there is **always** a valid explanation for why a child isn't sleeping. (There is more detailed information on sleep regressions in Chapter 3.)

Separation anxiety Many toddlers go through a degree of separation anxiety at some point, and it can be very challenging to manage. They can suddenly become clingy and cry when you leave the room, or not want to be held by anyone else. This can manifest further and cause problems at bedtime, when your toddler doesn't want you to leave the room. It's always important to understand what has sparked this change in behaviour and to work out the underlying cause so that you can address the issue, restoring the previous balance. Many older babies and toddlers who display separation-anxiety symptoms actually suffer from an underlying digestive discomfort that makes them crave their most trusted source of comfort, which is usually their mum, and when that comfort disappears it can upset them and bring on tears.

Nightmares and night terrors Many children experience nightmares and night terrors. Most will grow out of them and they won't cause any long-term psychological harm. Nightmares occur during REM, or 'dream', sleep, and your child may wake up from the nightmare and be able to remember and describe the dream to you. Night terrors are very different from nightmares; this behaviour occurs on waking abruptly from deep, non-dream sleep, and a child having night terrors may scream and thrash around, and may not recognize you if you try to comfort them. Your child won't be fully awake during these episodes, and will likely have no memory of them the next morning.

Acid-reflux and dietary issues Many parents have turned to me over the years for help with sleep-training their toddler. However, a large number of these toddlers don't need sleep-training but a change in diet and the effective management of a gastro-oesophageal reflux problem. The accepted ethos, that all babies grow out of 'colic' and acid-reflux by the time they are six or twelve months old, is a huge misconception; in my experience, it is one of the major factors contributing to the increase in cases of childhood sleep problems. Children who have heartburn from acid-reflux and/or digestive discomfort from an intolerance or allergy are not going to be able to sleep comfortably and will protest loudly when we try to make them! If this is an underlying problem then it is wholly inappropriate to implement any form of sleep-training until the issues have been fully and properly addressed, and you should first read Chapter 7 of this book to ensure you can rule out such problems.

Removing sleep-crutches

In my first book, *The Sensational Baby Sleep Plan*, as part of the reassurance sleep-training technique, I discuss removing 'sleep-crutches' – associations that a younger baby may have come to rely on for sleep, such as feeding to sleep, rocking or even full contact-sleep, where your baby will only sleep in your arms and not ever be put in a cot.

In the first few months of life, the environment you create to help your baby fall asleep will need to be recreated every time your baby then wakes or needs to settle back to sleep. For example, if you rock or feed your baby to sleep all the time, when your baby stirs through his natural sleep cycles, as is expected up to three or four months of age, he will wake and look for the same sensation to help settle him back to sleep, and therefore never learn to 'self-soothe'.

Many parents will reach a certain point in their baby's first twelve months when they decide to try to change the learned sleep associations, and thousands have successfully done so by following the reassurance sleep-training technique aimed at babies from the age of four months plus, as detailed in the first book. However, there are many other parents who haven't attempted to change things, because they either couldn't face doing so or were happy to leave things as they were, perhaps thinking their baby would grow out of their sleep-crutches. Whatever the reason, if you've reached twelve months or beyond and your toddler is still not sleeping or is needing contact and comforting to sleep, it's not too late to change things – but those associations and sleep-crutches will need to be removed as part of the reassurance sleep-training technique.

Please don't panic at this thought, though – it doesn't mean that you have to remove their beloved bunny or noo-noo. In fact, once they are near or past twelve months, it may be possible to give your toddler certain sleep comforts (for example, a special pillow or teddy) to replace the sleep-crutches (see p. 138). It's more about removing your own contact – whether that's holding their hand, rocking them, feeding them, sitting or lying next to them and letting them twirl your hair as they try to find sleep – and I'll be explaining exactly how to do this over the next two chapters.

The following is a list of the most common sleep-crutches that can become a hindrance to your toddler, and that will need to be addressed as part of sleep-training.

Feeding to sleep
This is such a common problem and an easy trap to fall into, as in the early weeks a baby can naturally fall asleep at the breast or while feeding from the bottle. If you haven't managed to change or stop this association during the first year, then it can prove to be a challenge, but it is certainly not impossible. When you implement reassurance sleep-training, you may still need to give your toddler a milk feed before he goes to bed, but you will need to ensure that he goes down awake, or at least drowsy – but certainly not fully asleep. If your child has been used to falling asleep while feeding then the prospect of putting him down awake may seem impossible, but hundreds of parents who have been in a similar situation now know it can be done, thanks to my sleep-training technique.

Night-time feeds
Most healthy babies do not really need night-time milk feeds after three months, and certainly by the age of one, two or three your child should be following their natural biological clock of the 12-hour split defined by day and night. Our digestive

systems are designed to take on food during the daylight hours, then digest, process, cleanse, rest and empty our systems throughout the night while we are sleeping, and expel the waste produced once we've woken in the morning. This simple yet scientifically proven process never seems to be attributed to older babies or toddlers as it is still deemed acceptable or normal for them to be having night-time milk feeds for months, if not years, on end! There really is no easy way to remove these night feeds other than by gradually reducing the volume you offer over a few days or else by just stopping – cold turkey!

The dummy
This is probably the most common sleep aid, but sadly it is often the biggest hindrance to sleep. Many parents find themselves getting up repeatedly throughout the night just to replace the dummy, and I have seen many babies systematically throw out every dummy in their cot, and then cry, in order to ensure a visit from Mum or Dad. Whether your toddler uses a dummy during the day, just at night or both, you have to remove it completely as it is unfair to expect her to learn to sleep without it if she is still allowed to use it for comfort during the day. (See p. 143 for how to remove the dummy for good.)

Contact-sleep strategies
Whether it's patting, rocking, stroking, hand-holding, cuddling or lying next to your toddler to get them to sleep, you will need to replace the 'contact' with reassurances that encourage your child to fall asleep by themselves. It can be incredibly challenging to stop these practices that your little one has become so used to, but by following the steps set out in Chapter 5 and implementing the reassurance technique, you will get there in the end.

Toddler sleeping in your bed

There are a number of scenarios surrounding co-sleeping – for example, your child starting off the night in her own bed and then creeping into yours during the night; you lying with him in your bed while he goes to sleep, then you leaving for a couple of hours before joining him when you go to bed; or perhaps your toddler stays up with you until you all go to bed together; or you may go to bed at 7pm with your toddler and stay with him all night! All these situations can be quite tricky to change, but by adapting the reassurance sleep-training technique accordingly, the situation can be resolved and your toddler will learn to love his own room and his own bed. It's never about just being 'tough' or putting him in his own room, closing the door and letting him get on with it – it's much more about working out how you've ended up co-sleeping, or part-co-sleeping, and planning how to adapt the reassurance sleep-training to meet your child's needs.

Delaying-tactics

This can be a challenging problem to resolve, particularly once a toddler can use words, as well as tears, to try to get you to stay with them. 'I'm scared' is a common cry and will definitely make your blood run cold; 'I need the toilet', 'I need another cuddle', 'I need some water' and 'I need a tissue' are just some examples of the delaying-tactics that your child may use to try to get you to stay longer in the room or keep re-visiting them. By setting firm boundaries, creating 'bedtime rules' and following all the steps in Chapter 5, you will be amazed at how quickly your little one responds and stops all the previous demands.

Hopefully you now feel somewhat more prepared and better equipped to manage your toddler's sleep-time behaviour, have everything you may need in place and have some help and support on-hand. You will have made sure there are no underlying digestive issues – or, if there are, you have them fully managed – and you now feel ready to go ahead and implement the reassurance sleep-training.

☆ ALISON'S GOLDEN RULES ☆

1. Be a 'baby detective' and first work out *why* your child is not sleeping.

2. Stop discussing the issues surrounding night-time and sleep within earshot of your toddler.

3. Prepare your child's bedroom for sleep-training, ensuring it is a safe environment, with no safety hazards.

4. Don't keep telling your child that things are going to change for days on end prior to implementing the changes as this could make them anxious about what's coming.

5. Ensure you've investigated and are successfully managing any acid-reflux, dietary intolerances or allergies, and changed your toddler's diet accordingly.

6. If your toddler has a dummy and you need to remove it, then have everything prepared to implement my dummy-removal method on the day you're going to start the sleep-training.

7. Enlist help from others – to look after other siblings, for example – so you can fully focus on the sleep-training.

8. Be prepared for the protests you are likely to encounter from your toddler and, difficult though this is, stay firm in your belief this will work and know that thousands of others have successfully followed the same technique.

9. Make sure any other adults who care for your child understand the method and have read this book so there is consistency and unity in your approach.

10. Put a bottle of wine, some beers or anything else you fancy on ice, ready to treat yourself once your toddler has gone to sleep – you will definitely deserve it!

CHAPTER 5

The Reassurance Sleep-training Technique

I have researched many methods of sleep-training, ranging from strict controlled crying to the more gentle approach of a 'no-cry' sleep solution. Having combined elements of various methods with my experience, expertise and understanding of babies and young children's sleep habits and requirements, along with my intuition, I have created my hugely popular reassurance sleep-training technique. Using various age-appropriate adaptations, this technique will work for babies from four months through to children up to four or even five years old. While in my first book, *The Sensational Baby Sleep Plan*, I explain how to use the technique for babies from four months through to older babies still in a cot, here I apply the technique to toddlers and young children and cover the sometimes tricky transition from cot to bed.

I have witnessed many distressing situations where families are getting little or no sleep each night, with seemingly little resolution on the horizon. Each week I receive many emails from desperate parents at the end of their tether and who feel I'm their 'last resort' as they've tried so many different things to get their child sleeping. Sleep deprivation is so debilitating, negatively affecting your mental and physical health, that after weeks of little or no sleep you simply don't have the energy to try to resolve things with your non-sleeping toddler. So, night after night, even though you want things to change, you just take the path of least resistance and continue to give a bottle of milk or to cuddle your little one to sleep, as you know by doing this you might yet get another 2 or 3 hours of sleep. The worry that things might get even worse if you do something different, and the possibility of failure in trying something new, is just unimaginable.

If any of this resonates, then please read on as my advice can, and will, work for your family too. So many parents before you have also felt the fear and faced, with trepidation, the thought that it won't work for them before finding the courage to embark on and implement the sleep-training.

THE BASIS OF REASSURANCE SLEEP-TRAINING

There are two underlying approaches you need to adopt that will lead to the success of this technique. These are: having an aura that exudes the 'Five Cs' and displaying behaviours in line with the 'Five Ps'. The Five Cs and Five Ps are as follows:

- Calm

- Controlled

- Confident

- Clear

- Consistent

- Plan

- Prepare

- Patience

- Persistence

- Perseverance

I fully appreciate that, deep down inside, you might be feeling a touch anxious, and while this is completely normal, now is the time you need to draw on your acting skills and portray a **calm** and **confident** outward expression and stay completely **controlled**. Children are innately in-tune with our moods and emotions, so the more you can adopt the 'Five Cs' ethos and hide your true feelings of angst, the better your toddler will respond. She will also be reassured by your **consistent** approach and your giving her one **clear** message: it's time to go to sleep!

Following the 'Five Ps' ethos, you will **plan** your strategy, be organized and fully **prepared**, then exert incredible **patience** throughout the entire time it takes to implement the sleep-training. You will need to find an inner strength, be **persistent** with the reassurances and **persevere** until your toddler realizes that you are not going to respond to his demands and decides to give up his protest before settling down to sleep.

It's not an easy process to go through sometimes, but if you can stick with the method, see it through and implement the technique as I describe it, it will bring huge rewards for you all.

PREPARING FOR REASSURANCE SLEEP-TRAINING

My reassurance sleep-training technique removes all previous uncertainty about sleep expectations, is easy to implement, sets clear boundaries for both you and your child – and has been proven successful time and time again.

Happily, the technique works in a relatively short space of time, which is another reason why it is so successful. As I explained in my first book, *The Sensational Baby Sleep Plan*, babies 'forget' learned associations within two to four days, and the new way you put your baby to bed – without rocking or patting, for example – quickly becomes the new norm. This is somewhat true for older babies and toddlers too, though the older they get, the longer their short-term memory becomes, so it can sometimes take two to three weeks to change the sleep associations of, say, a two- or three-year-old.

I often hear of parents who have been implementing some sort of sleep-training for much longer than a couple of weeks, and sometimes several months, which I believe is not only soul-destroying but, sadly, somewhat psychologically damaging to all involved.

> ### ALISON SAYS . . .
>
> 'If you follow my reassurance sleep-training technique, it really shouldn't take long before you see positive results. So many parents report back to me that it was so much easier than they imagined it would be and that they're utterly amazed at how quickly their little one responded.'

Health and safety guidelines

For many toddlers who do not sleep well, there is sometimes a more subtle, underlying cause that must be addressed before tackling any form of sleep-training. In fact, out of the thousands of parents who have contacted me asking for help with their little one's sleep, very few of these children actually have a genuine sleep disorder. Through in-depth consultation with the parents, I determine the child's history and glean details on many aspects of their health, daily routine, and what happened in the early weeks or months, to gain a clear understanding of the current situation and work out what could be the possible cause of the night-time wakings.

The following are just some of the questions I might ask and the reason why:

- *Question:* Did you have any complications in pregnancy?

  - ◆ *Reason:* A baby being premature, for example, may cause a slight developmental delay, which has affected longer-term sleep.

- *Question:* Has the child ever been exposed to antibiotics, either in utero, through breastfeeding or given directly?

  - ◆ *Reason:* It is a well-known fact that exposure of the immature gut to antibiotics can cause an intolerance to cow's-milk protein, and may give a clue why the toddler seems unable to sleep comfortably.

- *Question:* What milk are you currently giving? Breast milk or formula? If formula, which ones have you tried and which one do you give now? Are you using cow's milk or a plant-based alternative?

♦ *Reason:* Understanding the milk-feeding history helps build a picture of possible sleep-crutches or digestive causes for sleep problems. Is the toddler still reliant on breastfeeding to sleep, for example? If so, it may be due to reflux.

• *Question:* When did you introduce solids? Did it go well or was it tricky? What is your little one's attitude to food now? Are they a fussy eater, a snacker; perhaps they never sit still at mealtimes, or are constantly craving food and eating too much?

♦ *Reason:* Finding out what a child's eating habits are can reveal a lot about their digestion and gut health. If they are a particularly 'fussy' eater, it could mean they have acid-reflux. If they can't sit still for meals it can indicate that they are too uncomfortable to sit down for long periods. If they crave food and eat too much, it could mean they have learned to eat in response to digestive discomfort. This pain could explain why they are then unable to sleep at night.

• *Question:* Do they drink excessive amounts of water or refuse to drink much water at all?

♦ *Reason:* Drinking too much water can indicate that the toddler is trying to wash away burning pain from acid-reflux. Alternatively, a child may not want to drink water as it exacerbates a reflux issue, making him feel uncomfortable.

• *Question:* What is their poop history? (Colour, consistency, frequency . . .) Are they constipated, have loose stools, potty-trained or not? (NB: I often ask the client to send me a pic of their child's poop, so I can fully assess it for myself. The photo reel on my phone is not for the faint-hearted!)

- ◆ *Reason:* Much can be understood about gut health from a toddler's poop. For example, if they are constipated it could mean they have an intolerance to cow's-milk protein. If they have loose or mushy stools, it can indicate an intolerance to gluten. Any digestive discomfort will interfere with sleep.

- *Question:* What is the little one's skin like? Are there, or have there ever been, any rashes, allergic reactions, hives, spots, eczema or nappy rash?

  - ◆ *Reason:* Any skin rashes, eczema or spots can indicate a food intolerance or allergy and mean the child is too uncomfortable to sleep.

- *Question:* Have you noticed him pulling at his ears? Does he have waxy ears or scratch at his head?

  - ◆ *Reason:* Fluid can build up in the ear and cause pain when lying down. A sign of this can be excessive earwax.

- *Question:* Does he snore? Is he a 'mouth-breather'?

  - ◆ *Reason:* Many children who snore, breathe through their mouth when asleep or are very noisy breathers have an underlying acid-reflux issue that needs to be addressed before they can sleep properly.

- *Question:* Does he suffer with excessive bottom-wind and is it smelly? Does he ever seem to have a bloated, distended or swollen tummy?

◆ *Reason:* Excessive or smelly bottom-wind, along with a bloated tummy, can often indicate a food intolerance and cause much discomfort that impedes sleep.

- *Question:* What's his behaviour like?

  ◆ *Reason:* A toddler's behaviour can be very revealing. Aggressive play or hyperactivity, for example, can be caused by the child experiencing digestive pain due to some degree of intolerance or reflux issue.

- *Question:* Has anything unsettling, challenging or upsetting happened in the past few weeks or months?

  ◆ *Reason:* It's important to look at what has recently happened in your family life to see if there has been an unsettling event that may have triggered the night-time wakings.

- *Question:* What have you tried up to now to resolve the sleep issues? Were there any improvements or are things even worse?

  ◆ *Reason:* It's important to know if the child has been upset in any way from previous, unsuccessful sleep-training attempts, as we can then adapt the reassurance technique to ensure he has some added comfort while he learns to sleep.

Finding out the answers to all the above and more allows me to understand the bigger picture, and more often than not there are things that need addressing before we can even think about implementing any sleep-training. I've learned over the years that there is nearly always an underlying cause of sleep problems and on many occasions it is linked to the gut. I've often found there to be an undiagnosed acid-reflux problem that is still active and causing the child pain. Or there may be food intolerances and allergies that have not been recognized and that cause discomfort and tummy aches while the digestion process takes place throughout the night. These medical conditions often explain why a toddler is unable to sleep easily or has not responded well to any previous sleep-training. Of course, there are some scenarios that are purely behavioural and not linked to any medical issue, so I hope all the information set out in this book gives you the guidance you need to recognize if there may be a genuine underlying cause before implementing the sleep-training.

Always try to make sure that your child is fit and well before embarking on any form of sleep-training. It would be unfair to both you and your toddler to implement any changes if she were poorly and it would be better to wait a few days for the worst symptoms to pass and she was feeling well again. Obviously, some illnesses are not immediately apparent and may have an incubation period, so if you feel that your little one is even more unsettled or cranky than usual, it may be worth a trip to the GP to check there is no ear infection or other hard-to-spot ailment, before starting the sleep-training.

If your child is taken ill soon after implementing sleep-training, do not despair: although it may be a temporary setback, there is detailed information in the next chapters on how to manage this situation and get back on track.

Before sleep-training, it's vital you ensure your toddler will stay safe when left in his room. If he is still in a cot, ensure the base is at its lowest setting so he can't climb out, possibly falling in the process. If your toddler is showing signs of being able to climb out, even with the base at its lowest, or has already done so, then it is time to switch to a proper bed.

You can make a single or toddler bed safe quite easily by

first positioning it in a corner of the room, or at least longways against a wall, as the chances of falling off it are then halved. On the exposed side you can fit a foldable or inflatable bed-guard, and together these measures should prevent a tumble on to the floor.

Once your child moves into a bed, it's far better to provide a toddler duvet and pillow set instead of any previously used baby sleeping bag, as the restricted movement caused by the sleeping bag could prove to be a safety hazard. It is also advisable to check there are no potentially dangerous items in the bedroom that could cause your toddler serious harm. Remove or safeguard such items as an unstable wardrobe, chest of drawers or bookcase, loose blind or curtain cord, freestanding and accessible glass photograph frames or ornaments, and hot radiators, heaters or towel rails. Put child locks on windows to prevent them opening too far.

When suffering from sleep deprivation, some children can display quite aggressive behaviour, especially when you try to change things, such as their usual bedtime practices. Some can actually become quite destructive and throw their toys or belongings around the room in protest at the changes, or even resort to some degree of self-harm. Although this sounds utterly awful, it is more common than you might imagine and there is nearly always an underlying cause. In most cases it can be linked to a degree of undiagnosed and untreated acid-reflux that causes such discomfort to the child that he struggles to control his own feelings. This is why I always urge parents to work out if there are any underlying issues that could be the cause of the night-time wakings before embarking on full-blown sleep-training.

(NB: If your child does display the destructive and dangerous behaviours mentioned above, to keep him safe you may need to temporarily remove all toys, books and small furniture from his room.)

ALISON SAYS . . .

'I remember arriving at a house to help a family with their non-sleeping two-year-old, who was almost feral in his behaviour. Although the parents had insisted on the phone that there were no underlying reflux issues, as soon as I met the little boy I knew they were mistaken. He was food-phobic and couldn't sit still at mealtimes, was painfully thin although incredibly strong, and had speech delay. Although he only made noises, I could tell his "voice" was hoarse and croaky, which was due to damage from acid coming up from his stomach. He was so terrified of sleep, he became completely unmanageable when put in his bedroom, throwing his toys around the room and banging his head on the wall. He had a cabin bed that was positioned along a wall and partly covered a window, and within seconds he had climbed over to the other side of the bed and was clinging to the window frame, kicking the glass! And all this was just him showing me his room. I explained to the parents that I wasn't prepared to implement any form of sleep-training until we addressed his reflux issues and child-proofed his room. Two weeks later, with reflux symptoms under control through a dietary change and medicine prescribed by a paediatrician, I went back and was greeted with an almost completely different child! He was calm, had started to say words, had put on some weight and happily showed me his "new" and safer room. That night I instigated the "bedtime rules" (explained later in this chapter) along with my reassurance sleep-training, and within an hour – and with very little protest – he was asleep on his mattress on the floor and slept all night.'

A PARENT'S STORY

'Alison came to help with our five-month-old, but throughout her stay she not only improved things for our baby, she started asking questions about our two-year-old. He had always had "issues" with his behaviour, but we had been fobbed off by all the health professionals we had seen, who put it down to usual toddler behaviour. He had horrid poops that were mushy, runny and explosive, and we used to have to hose him down in the shower every time he did one. He constantly craved food and always overate. He seemed to have a permanent cough and cold and really waxy ears. Throughout the night, he produced so much mucus that his cot was soaked in the morning from thick saliva.

He was also very "highly strung" and sensitive, yet very loud, determined and stubborn, and seemed to have a very high pain threshold. We had managed to get him to accept going to bed for a daytime nap and at bedtime, but he would bang his head on the side of his cot for ages before eventually falling asleep. Nothing we did changed or prevented this behaviour and I used to cry almost every night listening to him. Alison was shocked and visibly distressed by what she witnessed, and then almost angry that no one had been able to help us. Alison knew all his behaviours were linked to his gut – and she was so right! It turned out he is gluten-intolerant, which was the main cause of all the problems, but he also had an active acid-reflux issue due to his gut not coping with what it couldn't digest. We removed gluten from his diet, treated his acid-reflux and, within days, along with all the symptoms subsiding, the head-banging stopped! Alison literally changed our lives and that of our two boys. I dread to think where it would have all ended up if we hadn't found her.'

E. H.

Preparing for sleep-training

As well as taking into account the safety guidelines set out above, you also need to consider the following points when preparing for sleep-training your toddler, because they, too, can affect the success of this technique:

Timing It is best to implement sleep-training when you have a clear diary, certainly without evening engagements, for a couple of weeks, so you can fully focus without interruption. It is also advisable to avoid starting sleep-training around the time of any disruptive events such as a vaccination, a holiday or your toddler beginning nursery, for example, any of which may have a negative effect on the process. That said, many parents have called me wanting to improve their little one's sleep, but with a holiday planned in the next few weeks, they think that it would be best to start sleep-training once they have returned. However, as long as there are at least ten days before your trip, it can be more beneficial to implement the changes before you go. Once children have settled into their new sleep pattern, understand what is expected of them and accept the 'new normal' for their night-time sleeping, they are usually quite adaptable to a change in environment or an hour-change, and having a sleep routine established before your holiday makes it easier to adapt when you travel. (There is more information on hour-changes and time-zone travel in Chapter 6.)

Unity It is essential that everyone involved with the care of your toddler understands how to use my sleep-training method, is fully committed to it and is prepared to provide as much support as possible throughout for the first few days and nights. Everyone must follow the same pattern and reinforce the 'sleepy-time' message, because if just one person decides to revert back to previous habits, it can cancel out all the effort and progress made up to that point and you'll have to start again.

Persevere However many times you may have tried, without success, to use sleep-training methods, it is vital that you find the strength and resolve to see my technique through. After so many failures, it may be hard to find the faith and to believe that this method will work, but I can assure you that it does. Very quickly you will begin to see positive improvements in your toddler's sleep, which in turn will give you the confidence to carry on. The more times you give up and try to restart, the more difficult it will become, because your toddler will quickly learn that there is still no consistency from one night to the next.

Siblings If your toddler shares a room with a sibling, either younger or older, if possible and just while you implement the technique, it might be helpful to move the other child to another room or even get them to stay with relatives or friends for a few nights. If, however, neither child who shares the room sleeps well, it is best to leave them together and carry out the sleep-training with them both at the same time. Likewise, if you have twins who share a room, it is fine to sleep-train them both together. Even if the siblings do not share rooms but both wake during the night, you can sleep-train them at the same time with them being in separate rooms.

Environment Make the bedroom as dark as possible and shield the natural morning light with heavy curtains or even a blackout blind, especially if your toddler is prone to early waking. Add a 'sleep-clock' that shows the difference between night and day and a dim-glowing night-light, give an extra teddy or other comforter, and play some white noise if it helps.

Routine As previously mentioned, it is important to put in place a good bath- and bedtime routine, which gives the signal that 'sleepy-time' is nearly here! Before bathtime, remember to try to instigate a lively and active half-hour that ends with 'tidy-up' time (see p. 89). Then, after a fun bathtime, you can start to create the calmer atmosphere needed for the short period before bed, with two or three stories, for example, followed by milk, teeth-cleaning, a song, cuddles and kisses before tucking them up in bed.

De-sensationalize Prior to embarking on the sleep-training, avoid constantly talking about the 'sleep problem' with other family members or having a long discussion about it with a friend, especially when your toddler is within earshot – if you do need to discuss things with another adult, then wait until your toddler is playing in the garden, upstairs in bed or perhaps at nursery. Even though the sleep issues have been plaguing your life and it's all you can think about, you need to try to de-sensationalize the situation and keep things happy and calm within the home. The more your child hears you talking about the night-time problems, the more likely you'll heighten her awareness that night-time is a huge problem, and her anxiety will continue to build, which will make it much harder to implement the necessary changes.

Don't involve your child Many parents make the mistake of involving their toddler in preparing for the imminent changes to their sleeping routine – for example, by taking them to choose a bed and a new duvet set. While children need to be involved in certain aspects of family and daily life, so they feel included, it's best to avoid creating a big fuss around implementing sleep-training as it simply causes your child to become more anxious about it. Although she may seem excited about her new bed and may not fully understand what's about to happen, she will still be having feelings of anxiety about the impending changes that continue to gain traction the more you talk about it.

SETTING THE SCENE

Being properly prepared before implementing the reassurance technique itself will ensure a smoother transition through the necessary changes.

Substituting sleep-crutches

In Chapter 4 I detailed all the sleep associations that need to be stopped or changed, or for which you could provide some substitute distraction or reassurance. Below are several substitutes you could use; you can choose to give either one or more – whatever you think your toddler will enjoy or respond to, and will therefore help with the imminent changes.

A cuddly toy or comforter If your toddler already has a special muslin, 'blankie', favourite cuddly toy or other comforter that they sleep with, it's fine to let them keep using it; if they don't already have one, you might want to introduce one as replacement comfort when ceasing your sleep-time cuddles or removing the dummy, for example. However, it's important that you instil some rules around its use and do not let it interfere with the sleep-training process. For example, if after bedtime your child throws the comforter to the floor, you need to leave it where it landed and not give it back when you enter the room to deliver reassurance. Even if your child cries and pleads with you to give it back to them, I'm afraid you must ignore their demands and carry on with your cool and confident reassurances. In the morning, when you get your little one up for the day, you can pick up the comforter – or encourage him to do so himself – and put it back in his cot or bed. He will learn very quickly that if he wants his beloved doggy with him at night then he should not throw it out! Equally, if your child is still clinging to his comforter when you get him up in the morning, then you need to encourage him to leave the comforter in the cot or bed and not to take it downstairs. These comforters are for sleep-time use only and it will become something positive to be looked forward to as sleep-time approaches.

Night-light As children get older, many of them seem to need a light, which helps to comfort them throughout the night. Choose one that gives just a soft glow rather than a really bright light, and make sure it is not a 'blue light' of any kind. I have also found that some toddlers can be calmed and distracted at bedtime by using a rotating disco ball or light-show lamp that projects images or lights on to the ceiling, but of course these need to be turned off when it is actually bedtime.

Sleep-clock There are a number of sleep-clocks on the market, but I particularly like the Groclock, made by the Gro Company. This is a programmable clock that will show a yellow sun-face during the day and display a blue, sleeping star-face through the hours of the night, so even very young children, not yet able to tell the time, can tell when it's awake-time or sleepy-time. Though marketed for use with children aged two years and above, I have successfully used such clocks for babies as young as ten months and they are particularly useful for combating early-morning waking. What is vital is understanding how to use them effectively. For example, if you've set the clock to indicate the awake-time from 6.30am and your toddler wakes before this time, put her back to bed if she gets out, and ensure her day doesn't start until the sun comes up on the clock. Some sleep-clocks also double as a night-light, if your child likes to have a light on in her room throughout the night, with variable brightness at different times of the night.

White noise I have found that using white noise can often help older babies and toddlers settle more easily and sleep more deeply. Importantly, white noise needs to be played for the full duration of a nap and all through the night. There are many white-noise products that you can turn on at bedtime but which will then play for only 20–40 minutes; this actually interferes with sleep and encourages your little one to wake after a sleep cycle, rather than settling the child and linking sleep cycles together. So, make sure you have the noise playing on a loop through a smart-speaker or buy an actual white-noise machine that plays continually.

Audio-stories For some toddlers who struggle to fall asleep at bedtime, an audio-story can be helpful to listen to once they are in bed. However, you will need to monitor your child's behaviour while the story is playing. For example, if he gets up, is shouting or messing around and not really listening to the story, turn it off and carry out your 'goodnight' routine, followed by the reassurances as described later in this chapter.

ALISON SAYS . . .

'An idea I came up with some time ago that can really help when removing a toddler's need for your physical contact in order to fall asleep is to have one or more photographs of yourself printed on to a pillow case, or a small cushion, and give it to your toddler at bedtime as a comforting replacement for your physical presence so they still have "you" to cuddle when going to sleep. I call it a Mummy or Daddy pillow or refer to it as their "cuddle-cushion".'

The Magic Sleep Fairy's bedtime rules

My 'bedtime rules' are an incredibly useful tool to assist with the sleep-training process and will give your toddler a clear explanation of what is expected from them at bedtime and throughout the night, removing all previous chaos and confusion. The rules are not essential to sleep-training, though, and if you would prefer not to use them simply follow all the preparation guidelines and implement the technique as detailed but without devising or referring to the 'bedtime rules'.

I devised the rules years ago and have used variations of them with thousands of toddlers. Many parents have followed my advice and successfully created their own rules for their children. Typically, I use the rules for children aged eighteen months and up, and if you feel your little one will understand the concept, here's how to create them.

On a poster-size piece of card or paper write the heading 'The Magic Sleep Fairy's Bedtime Rules' or you can personalize it with your child's name, such as 'Amelia's New Bedtime Rules'.

If you're creating the rules for a toddler and have a baby sleeping in his own room, you must use the names of both children, e.g. 'Amelia and Adam's New Bedtime Rules', so your toddler doesn't feel as though she is being singled out.

Write your rules under the heading, across the top half of the paper. Your rules need to state what you're changing or implementing, and you can make them specific to your own situation, as required. Below are two examples of rules you might write on their poster:

Example 1

1. After your milk, two stories and some kisses and cuddles, it will be time to get into bed.

2. You have your water, a hankie and your bunny, which is everything you need for your night-time.

3. After bedtime, the lights will be turned off and the bedroom door closed.

4. You have your nappy on throughout the night so there's no need for you to get up for the toilet.

5. Everyone sleeps in their own bed and stays in their own room throughout the night.

6. You need to stay in bed until we come and get you up when it's morning.

Example 2

1. After your stories at bedtime, the yellow sun-face will go to sleep on the 'magic clock' to show you it's sleepy-time.

2. Once the magic clock is blue, you will know it is sleepy-time and Mummy/Daddy will leave the room so you can go to sleep.

3. All lights go off when it's sleepy-time, except the blue star-face on the magic clock, and the bedroom door must stay closed.

4. All through the night and while the magic clock is blue, you must stay in your own bed in your own room.

5. In the morning, you can only get out of bed when the yellow sun-face comes up on the magic clock, and Mummy or Daddy comes in to get you.

Once you've devised and written up your rules, engage your child with decorating the bottom part of the poster. Give him some special stickers to use, perhaps cut out some pictures or use photos of family members that he can stick on, or let him use some crayons or paints to embellish the poster (obviously, don't let him cover the rules you have written with his 'decorations'). It is important that you engage him with decorating the poster, even if in just a small way, as this makes the rules more personal to him and he will feel a sense of 'ownership' towards the poster. Now read the rules to him, just once, and explain they are going to be put up in his bedroom. If your child gets upset about the rules, try to distract him, divert his focus and don't engage in a heated discussion with him about them. Just finish the decorating and put the poster up in his bedroom, somewhere out of reach.

Make the bedtime rules in the afternoon of the day you've chosen to start implementing the sleep-training and put them up in your toddler's room so they're ready for bedtime.

Reading aloud the rules, at some point before settling your child into bed, will now become part of your bedtime routine. Try to involve him when you do this; ask him if he remembers what the rules say and talk about the lovely decorations he has added. Even if he gets upset when you read the rule that says Mummy will leave the room, for example, try to ignore his cries and carry on reading them. Once you have read them, it will be bedtime and you will continue to implement the reassurance sleep-training from that moment onwards.

Removing the dummy

The method I use to successfully remove the dummy is easy to implement, fun and interactive but leaves your child with a clear understanding that their dummy has gone for good. Removing it may seem to be an absolute impossibility and fill you with utter dread, but it can be done and nearly always turns out to be less stressful than you first imagine.

When dealing with toddlers, it is better for them to view this as a normal progression and a natural part of growing up rather than a sensational, anxiety-filled event that causes much upheaval in their lives. Leading up to the day you have set to remove the dummy and start sleep-training, casually mention, and bring briefly into conversation now and again, that your toddler really no longer needs their dummy. Some toddlers may challenge you on this and you will need to be prepared with a reason why they can't have their dummy any more. It is quite likely they may not want to listen, but a reason still needs to be given just the same.

Depending on your child's age and personality, and their level of understanding, you could choose one or two of the following reasons (or make up your own):

- 'Now you have reached two years old, it means it is time to give up your dummy.'

- 'The dentist has said you need to stop sucking on your dummy as it might make your teeth wonky.'

- 'You often have your dummy in your mouth when you talk, and this means you always sound funny.'

- 'You had a message from the Dummy Fairy, who has said it is time for you to send her your dummy.'

The most important thing your child needs to know is the fact that all their dummies, some time soon, are going to be sent to the 'Magic Dummy Fairy'!

It's difficult to know how the individual child is going to respond when being told that their treasured dummy is going to be sent away for ever, and it is important to find the right balance between allowing discussion of the subject and ignoring any outright refusals and arguments. Some conversation and questioning is to be expected, but it is best to change the subject and use any number of distraction techniques if your child begins to cry and gets very upset. Of course they might not like to hear about the impending plan to remove the dummy, and some children may become easily disturbed at the thought of it, so in the end the decision about how to handle the preparation process, and how much prior information you give, will be up to you.

The dummy hunt
On the chosen day, you will need to have ready a large envelope or Jiffy bag and some special stickers, and to make a note of where all the dummies in the house are located (or purposely place them ready to be 'found'). Next you need to involve your child with decorating the envelope into which all the dummies will be put. You can allow any amount of stickers, colouring or drawing and address the envelope to:

The Magic Dummy Fairy

Dummy Land

The World

Then send your child (or children) on 'The Great Dummy Hunt' around the house to collect all the dummies. Once collected, encourage your child to put the dummies into the envelope and seal it up quickly. Then head off to the nearest post box as soon as possible, where you will need to encourage the child to post the envelope themselves while saying 'goodbye' to their dummies. Even though your child may be crying and very upset at 'posting' his beloved dummies, try not to worry and keep yourself calm while trying to distract your little one. You could head to a nearby park and hope that some outdoor fun will help him forget about his dummies or, once back home, find some engaging activity that will distract him.

NB: In order to avoid actually putting waste items into the

post box, add the appropriate stamps and post the envelope to the address of a family member or friend (not to yourself), then when the envelope arrives the dummies can be disposed of without your child ever seeing them. Alternatively, see the 'Dummy Fairy pack' available on my website that includes an envelope pre-addressed to me; I send some of the dummies for reuse on farms, where they help stimulate the sucking reflex in orphaned lambs.

Involving your toddler in the whole process of taking away the dummy actually brings its own rewards because your child has full knowledge of what has happened to his dummies and many never actually ask for one again. Some children do continue to ask to have their dummy back but, once reminded where the dummies have gone, will usually accept the situation without much fuss or further questioning. Undoubtedly there will be some children who will be inconsolable and have a problem accepting the situation, and if you believe your child may fall into this category it would be a good idea to have a special gift that has come from 'the Magic Dummy Fairy', which you can give at an appropriate moment to try to placate your upset child.

The rest of the afternoon will hopefully pass quite smoothly and without too much upset, but if your child has been reliant on his dummy to sleep with at bedtime, then there will very likely be more tears, demands to have his dummy back and a refusal to go to bed without it! If this happens, stay calm and try to distract him by reminding him of the new bedtime rules that he has decorated and showing him the other sleep comforters you may have put in place, such as a cuddle-cushion, a new night-time teddy or the sleep-clock, and follow through with implementing the full reassurance sleep-training as you put him to bed.

Transition from cot to bed

Firstly, don't sensationalize the fact that your little one has a new bed. Just keep it all low-key and treat it as a totally normal experience that every child goes through. On the day you are going to implement the sleep-training, get the new bed set up in your child's bedroom and child-proof the room as explained on p. 131.

If your child has a dummy, you could leave the dummy in place for a few days and remove it once she has got used to the transition from cot to bed, but ultimately it is better to remove the dummy on the day you implement sleep-training or as soon as you can face it!

I advise putting a sleep-clock in place alongside the bedtime rules when you make the transition from the cot, as these two things give your toddler some very clear guidelines about staying in bed and not getting out of her bed until morning.

Now, carry out your normal bath- and bedtime routine, and try not to let your little one jump all over her new bed. She may be excited about the new addition to her room and some inquisitive exploration is acceptable, but you do need to remind her that it is a place to sleep and not to play. Once you have finished story-time and she has had her milk, cleaned her teeth and read the bedtime rules, after some lovely cuddles and kisses you say your 'goodnights', settle her into the new bed and leave the room.

Close the door and wait to see what happens. It is highly possible she will stay in bed and go to sleep, but equally feasible she will get out of bed and come to the door. (It is of course easier to monitor the situation if you have a video camera strategically placed in the room so you can see what she's up to.) If she does get up, is crying or not going to sleep, then you will need to return to the room to deliver the reassurances as part of the sleep-training technique and persevere until she stays in bed and goes to sleep.

ALISON SAYS . . .

'Over many years I have worked with many families from different cultures, backgrounds, religions and countries. One very interesting experience was with a South African family who had never used a Moses basket, crib or cot. Instead, they put their baby to sleep in a toddler-size truckle bed. The family had two older daughters, both of whom had used this bed from birth and had then been moved into an ordinary single bed when they were around eighteen months old. Interestingly, even when the babies had got older, become more mobile, could crawl and walk, they had never got out of this little truckle bed during the night, and they moved to a big bed without any issues. Changing to a big bed was accepted as a normal phase by the children, as opposed to the often fraught and overcomplicated life event it seems to have become for many parents and their children today.

With my knowledge of toddler behaviour and developmental milestones, I often advise parents to put toddlers into a proper bed – or take the side off the cot – sooner rather than later, with remarkable success. I now believe the optimum age to do this is between eighteen and twenty-four months.'

A PARENT'S STORY

'My twin boys, River and Tristan, had just turned twenty months old when they became too big for their cots. I'm Alison's niece and, thanks to having Alison's help from very early on, the boys had always been great sleepers – from around twelve weeks old they had slept for 12 hours most nights, along with having good naps in the day – so I was reluctant to change anything and was nervous that switching them to proper beds, as Alison had advised, would undo all their fabulous sleep habits. However, I took the plunge and on the first night, after about ten re-visits to shoo them back to bed and reiterate my "sleepy-time" reassurances, they went to sleep! The second night I only had to go in twice and, ever since, bedtime has continued to pass without any issues. They also nap beautifully in their big beds and still sleep 11–12 hours each night. My fear of change, I now know, was wholly unfounded.'

C. I.

USING THE TECHNIQUE

This technique comprises setting clear boundaries, staying firm and resolute in your approach, implementing a calm and practical bedtime routine, monitoring your child after bedtime and responding appropriately with visits back into the room to deliver the reassurances – the 'sleepy-time' messages – and encourage your toddler to self-settle for sleep. The 'reassurances' are designed to do exactly that – to 'reassure' your little one. He might be upset at the changes you've put in place and may well be crying in protest, but rather than just closing the door and letting him 'cry it out', I feel it is far more appropriate for him to know you are still there and to benefit from your presence in his room, albeit at brief intervals. I know you will be asking when to go in, when to wait, what to say and what to do, and all is explained in detail throughout the rest of this chapter.

When the day you've chosen to start sleep-training has arrived, by following the 'Five Ps' ethos you should at least feel prepared and have a plan. I'm sure you will have a certain amount of trepidation at the thought of what's to come, but try to remember to adopt the 'Five Cs' and stay as calm and controlled as possible.

Once you have carried out your bath- and bedtime routine, read the bedtime rules, set the sleep-clock (if using one), introduced any new sleep-comforts you've provided and settled your little one into bed, it is time to leave the room.

As you leave the room, say to him, 'Goodnight, Hugo, it's sleepy-time now', or devise a similar short, basic phrase that you prefer – just make sure you include these words with whatever else you say to your child throughout the sleep-training process and beyond. Ensure that anyone else involved in helping you says the same thing. In multilingual families it is best if the phrase is said in the mother's language first, and then repeated in the second language, during each reassurance visit to settle your child. I like phrases that incorporate 'It's sleepy-time' as I find this easily becomes the focal point that doesn't change, whatever else I might say. For example, every time I re-enter the room to resettle him I will say, 'That's enough now, Hugo. It's sleepy-time. Night-night.' Or, if I have made the transition from cot to bed and the child has got out of bed, when I re-enter the room I will say, 'Get back into bed, Hugo. It's sleepy-time.' As you say goodnight to your child and put him in his cot or bed, you might repeat your chosen phrase a few times, always making sure your voice is calm, confident and reassuring.

Where possible, try to make it a bedtime rule that your toddler's bedroom door is closed, as I feel it reinforces the clear boundary between day and night, which allows the child to sleep better in their room without listening to noises from the rest of the house. That said, if you genuinely feel your toddler responds better to having the door ajar, then you can leave it open a little way.

If your toddler is still crying after a number of minutes, you will then have to go back into the room to deliver your 'sleepy-time' message, adding words to your basic phrase, such as, 'That's enough now', if he's crying, or 'Get back to bed', saying it in a much firmer tone of voice to convey that you are in control, you mean business and are no longer a soft touch! It can be hard to believe, but your child will respond and react more positively if you sound firm and in control than if you try to whisper softly or use a meek and mild voice. A soft, hesitant tone can instigate feelings of insecurity and uncertainty, whereas he will be more comforted and reassured by Mummy sounding confident, firm and in control, even if you don't feel that you are. Remember the 'Five Cs'!

If the crying continues, you will periodically need to keep re-visiting the room and reinforcing your sleepy-time message, until the crying has subsided, stopped or your toddler has gone to sleep. Whether you need to lay him back down, put him back on the bed, offer a few reassuring pats or, ideally, refrain from much physical contact, will be explained further on.

When using the reassurance sleep-training technique, parents always ask how long they should wait before going back in after putting the toddler to bed, and then how much time to leave between visits back into the room. I'm afraid there is no standard time-frame to follow. You have to decide for yourselves when it is necessary to re-visit the room, to speak through the monitor or to go in and stay in the room for a while. If your toddler is really crying, you might go in and out every few minutes; if he's just moaning and whingeing, you wouldn't need to visit at all. The 'Toddler Tears and Tantrums' table on p. 172 should also help you to judge how to respond.

ADAPTING THE TECHNIQUE TO YOUR NEEDS

The technique is designed to be somewhat flexible and can be adapted to better fit your specific situation, altered to be appropriate for a different age range and tweaked to best match the individual needs of your toddler. Whatever the scenario you face with your little one, with a few adjustments to the technique your situation can be changed and sleep, peace and harmony restored to your household.

Whether you choose to start the sleep-training with a daytime nap or at bedtime is up to you (and, of course, depends on whether your child still has a daytime nap). With older babies and toddlers I usually find it is better to start at bedtime, continuing with the technique throughout the night to manage any night-time wakings and using the same method for any daytime nap. That said, sometimes it's easier, and can relieve some of the intensity, to focus just on the nights at first, then applying it to the naps a few days later.

There are many different scenarios that will require individual adaptations of the technique, and you will need to decide when this is the best course of action for your little one. For example:

- Perhaps your toddler is still in a cot and not ready to move to a bed.

- You may decide to adapt the sleep-training to incorporate the transition from the cot to the bed – or from your bed into your child's own bed and room.

- Some toddlers like to have a teddy to cuddle, whereas others do not feel any benefit from a comforter at all.

- In some situations it is helpful to introduce a 'sleep-clock' that shows toddlers the time in a way they understand.

- If you are dealing with 'dummy removal' while sleep-training, you will need to adapt the method accordingly.

- Some children respond well to the 'sleepy-time' message, while others seem to get upset by it.

- It may be just the daytime nap that you need to establish, as your little one sleeps well at night, or you may need to use the technique for both day- and night-time sleep.

- Many children seem to feel reassured by sharing a room with a sibling, but others do better in a separate bedroom.

- It may not be bedtime that's the problem with your toddler, but that she wakes up in the middle of the night and comes into your bed, refusing to stay in her own.

- You may have to wean your toddler off night-time feeding, either gradually reducing the amount offered or going cold turkey.

- It could be a complete bedtime refusal you are dealing with, and your child resists ever being put to bed.

- Maybe your toddler goes to bed fairly easily, but stays awake for ages before they seem able to fall asleep.

- It might be an early waking problem that you need to address.

- Your toddler might be head-banging, scratching himself or causing some other degree of 'self-harm'.

- Perhaps your toddler appears to sleep OK but always seems restless, hot and sweaty while asleep and often wakes in the night, not getting the quality of sleep she needs.

The following is a detailed example of my 'hands-on' experience that shows how I created and used bedtime rules, removed dummies and implemented my reassurance sleep-training technique . . . with twins! By following all the advice given throughout this book, you too can create your own 'sleep-success story', just as I did – and that was while under the pressure of having a TV camera-crew watching my every move!

Back in 2010, I was asked to take part in a Channel 4 television programme called *Who Knows Best: Can't Sleep Kids*. The show set two sleep specialists head-to-head to see whose method proved best. I was introduced to a lovely mum called Susie with twenty-two-month-old twins, who were to be my 'challenge'. Poppy and Thomas shared a small bedroom, were still in cots, were addicted to endless bottles of milk throughout the night and attached to their beloved dummies, all of which meant there was little sleep to be had each night, for anyone.

I decided to put toddler beds in place, with duvets and pillows, and child-proof their bedroom, then stop giving bottles of milk in the night and remove the dummies – yup, all in one go! So we got everything organized and the afternoon before the first night I instigated the 'dummy hunt', taking the twins to post their envelopes full of dummies. There was some protest, but they were soon distracted with a session on some park swings on the way back home. I then created a poster on which I wrote some bedtime rules, and after helping both Poppy and Thomas to add some decoration, I put the poster up, out of reach, in their bedroom.

As bath- and bedtime approached, Susie was beside herself with anxiety, unable to believe the twins would ever go to sleep and certain they would just scream in response to all the changes. After stories, bedtime milk and reading out the bedtime rules, I put the twins into bed at 7.15pm. It took until 9.20pm for them to go to sleep! During those two hours, they cried, got out of bed countless times, shouted for more milk and pleaded for the long-gone dummies. At one point, they even tried to swap pyjamas! Once they had gone to sleep, however, we didn't hear another peep from them until nearly 7am. Susie hadn't slept all night, expecting them to wake at any moment, but they never did. And although the bedtime antics carried on for a few more nights, within a week the novelty had worn off and they happily settled each night and slept through!

Susie described herself as having been like a 'total robot' during those nights with the twins before we changed things. She said it felt like she just switched to autopilot, and as soon as either of them would wake she would go in, give them back the dummy that had been thrown on the floor, and if they still didn't sleep, she would resort to a bottle of milk – and this happened at least three or four times every night. She explained that, although she knew they didn't need the milk, she knew that they would sleep for an hour or so after having it and that was better than no sleep at all. I'm still in touch with Susie and she still has my name saved in her phone as 'Alison My Saviour' – which we still laugh about today!

Taking part in the show was a fantastic experience and, as it was set up as a competition, you might want to know who was the winner . . . Yes – you guessed right – it was me, the Magic Sleep Fairy. The twins pretty much slept through from night three, but at the end of the challenge the two-year-old whom my 'opponent' was working with was sadly still waking multiple times each night.

Sleep-training toddlers still in a cot

Babies aged twelve months or more can prove to be a little more resistant to sleep-training than younger babies as their learned habits and sleep associations are more deeply ingrained, so it takes longer for them to adapt and accept change. Your baby will also be more mobile and be able to sit or stand up in her cot, so you will need to firmly lay her back down at the same time as you deliver your 'sleepy-time' phrase. Often, before you even get to the door she will be standing up again, but you need to ignore her and continue to leave the room, then shut the door behind you. If she sounds as though she is standing again and is crying out or shouting, re-visit a few minutes later, repeating the same process. If she is standing up but not crying, or sitting or lying down and fairly quiet, then just wait and do not re-visit. You need go back in only if the level of cry or distress is building and you feel the need to give another reassurance. Otherwise just sit and wait to see what she does. If the crying escalates, go back in and continue to give reassurances, but if she is just moaning, chatting or crying at a low level then just wait and see if she settles down by herself.

It is helpful to mix up your reassurances by sometimes not going into the room at all and delivering the sleepy-time message through the closed door or a two-way sound monitor. Other times you might go into the room, stay completely quiet and not say anything at all, but simply prise her hands off the side of the cot, lay her down and then leave the room. Sometimes it's helpful to repeat visits a number of times in fairly quick succession and then leave her for perhaps 10 minutes before re-visiting the room and delivering another reassurance if she is still crying.

If she has thrown her bunny, teddy or comforter out of the cot, leave it on the floor where she threw it, though you might decide to hand it back to her the first time – if so, make sure you say, 'Here's Bunny back, but if he goes on the floor again he will stay there! Now it's sleepy-time. Night-night.' If Bunny gets thrown out a second time then you *must* ignore it and Bunny, I'm afraid, will need to stay on the floor until morning. I doubt, after that first night, her beloved bunny will ever be thrown out again!

You will quickly learn what your little one responds to positively and what seems to upset her more. For example, some toddlers seem to get angrier when the chosen phrase is used and are calmer when they are laid down without being spoken to. Others will immediately stop crying when the phrase is delivered and stay quiet for longer, and sadly some will just get upset whatever you do!

It is fascinating to watch through a video camera how a toddler's reaction changes to the sleep-training process as things progress. To start with, they may be continually standing up and even shaking the bars of the cot with utter frustration, shouting at the tops of their voices. Although the level of their cry can sound absolutely heartbreaking, I've often watched as they stop for a few moments and listen to see if they can hear you moving around, then ramp up the crying again. Usually, after a while they run out of steam and can only manage a sitting position, from which they eventually give in and lie down to sleep. I've witnessed many toddlers actually fall asleep in the sitting position before allowing themselves to actually lie down. It will be tempting to go in and lay them down, but I would advise leaving them to work it out for themselves – unless, of course, you're worried they may bang their head. If this is a possibility, it's a good idea to fit some padded cot bumpers, which will prevent any bumps and bruises. (NB: The World Health Organization guidelines on safe sleeping for your baby state: 'Keep your baby's sleep area (for example, a crib or bassinet) in the same room where you sleep until your baby is at least six months old, or ideally, until your baby is one year old. Keep soft bedding such as blankets, pillows, bumper pads and soft toys out of your baby's sleep area.' Considering my sleep-training is devised for babies aged twelve months and over, one can deem it safe to give your toddler a comforter or soft toy, and to fit cot bumpers if necessary. However, you can always put an under-mattress breathing sensor in place for added peace of mind.)

During the months that your baby is still in a cot, it's likely that her vocabulary will increase. As she learns more words it can become increasingly difficult to ignore her pleas, cries and demands. However, it is really important that you try not to respond to the words and just reinforce your sleepy-time phrase. Remember that the process will be more effective if you ignore the demands and questions, and carry on delivering the sleepy-time reassurances – quite simply, 'It's *sleepy-time*', and not time for conversation or discussions! That said, you will need to make a judgement on what to respond to and what to ignore. For example, you might allow them to tell you what they are desperate to divulge by saying 'OK, I'm listening, tell me what you need and then it will be sleepy-time.' Often, not much information will be forthcoming as your toddler didn't really have anything to tell you in the first place, but whatever it is she imparts, you must simply respond with something like 'OK, thank you for telling me. There's nothing to worry about right now and we can discuss it all in the morning as it's now *sleepy-time*!'

Ideally your toddler will be in his own room, but if limited space means he is still in a cot in your room, then you can still successfully carry out the sleep-training. Try to move the cot into a corner of your room, as far away from your bed as possible, and perhaps arrange things so he can't see you or your bed by using full-size cot bumpers, a room divider or even a curtain to section off his area. White noise can be useful in this situation too as it will help drown out any noise you make when going to bed or during the night, but it means you've got to get used to sleeping with it on too! It might be an idea to move out of your room for a few nights and 'camp out' in the living room while you implement the changes, then move back in once your child is routinely sleeping well.

SLEEP-TRAINING TODDLERS IN A BED OR TRANSFERRING TO ONE

The only real difference when your toddler is in a bed is that they can get out, being no longer restrained by the bars of the cot, so you do need to be mindful of the safety guidelines (see p. 131). Whether it's the first night of the new bed or you made the transition some time ago, the way to manage bedtime refusal or night-time wakings is almost the same and you will need to use the reassurance sleep-training technique for both.

ALISON SAYS . . .

'Many parents feel quite apprehensive about transitioning their toddler to a bed as they are convinced they will be up all night with their toddler roaming free, but in reality this is rarely the case – especially if you're following my advice! I always tell parents that when you remove the cot bars you need to replace them with effective parenting, through putting boundaries and rules firmly in place.'

Once you've finished your usual bath- and bedtime routine, or devised one following my earlier advice as part of the sleep-training technique, settle your child into her bed. She may already be tucked up in bed while you read bedtime stories either sitting on the floor or cuddling on the bed with her, but as soon as stories are finished you need to read the bedtime rules, if you didn't do so before story-time, and then after good-night kisses and cuddles get up and leave the room.

Be careful with the snuggling at story-time if your little one has been used to you lying with her while she goes to sleep; although you want to have closeness and cuddles while reading, it is unfair to lie with her as she may think you're going to stay while she sleeps. You may need to change the story-time environment and perhaps sit together on a beanbag or sofa in her room; sitting by her on the floor may also be effective. Once story-time has finished, settle her into bed on her own after your goodnight, hugs and cuddles. Equally, if your toddler is used to sleeping in your bed for either part or all of the night, your bedroom needs to become 'out of bounds'. It would be unwise to host story-time on your bed, then try to make her go to her own room, as she is likely to get more upset. It is kinder to completely remove the sleep association with your bed and bedroom.

You will have turned on the sleep-clock or night-light, if using one, started the white noise, made sure she has her cuddle-cushion, bunny and drink of water etc. Upon leaving the room, close the door behind you . . . and wait to see what happens. Watch on the video monitor if you have one.

It is likely she will start crying and get out of bed, and you will need to use your reassurance phrase whether she is sitting in bed, crying or has got out of bed. If she does get up and approaches the door, go straight back in and tell her firmly to get back to bed. Try to 'herd' her across the room, 'shooing' her back to the bed and encouraging her to get on to and into the bed herself, rather than picking her up, giving cuddles and tucking her back in. If she won't go to the bed on her own, take her hand, lead her across the room and, if nothing else works, pick her up – but just deposit her on the bed while telling her it's sleepy-time. Then turn away, walk out and deliver the sleepy-time message.

The thing to understand here is that it might seem harsh not to sit with her and tuck her back into bed, but you already did that – at bedtime. It's not bedtime now, it's sleepy-time, and if she chooses to get out of bed after her lovely, comforting bedtime, then she has to learn that there are consequences to this and she will need to settle herself back to bed on her own. Sometimes there will be huge protests and copious tears, and she may try to cling on to you, which is obviously distressing. You must try to stay calm, extricate yourself from her as quickly as you can and leave the room. No matter how many times she gets up and comes to the door or out of the room, repeat the same process and keep putting her back until she decides to stay put and go to sleep.

While implementing the technique, you still need only deliver sleepy-time messages such as 'That's enough, Sarina. It's sleepy-time' or 'Get back to bed, Sarina. It's still sleepy-time.' If you have left her with a dummy and she throws it out or has 'lost' it, if she demands more cuddles, books, kisses, water or milk, for example, you must ignore this and carry on with delivering the same bedtime phrase and putting her back to bed every time she gets up. During the night, any time she wakes up, cries out or gets out of bed, repeat the above and stick with it till morning.

By the time you've decided to put your toddler into a bed or are addressing sleep issues for an older child, the vocabulary development is likely to have been substantial and your little one can probably use a whole sentence or three. This can make the sleep-training more difficult as it will be harder to ignore their demands and to stick to just delivering the sleepy-time message rather than engage in conversation.

Over the years, along with the more usual cries of feeling unwell, scared, hungry, thirsty, needing a cuddle, etc., I've heard many clever things said by toddlers to get some reaction. Some examples I've heard are:

- 'I'm going to tell Daddy/Grandma that you're being horrid.'

- 'I will stop crying if you sit with me.'

- 'I'm going to cry *all* night and never go to sleep.'

- 'Please don't shut the door. If you leave it open I will stop crying.'

- 'What are we doing tomorrow, Mummy?'

- 'What's for breakfast tomorrow?'

- 'I *really* need to tell you something.'

If your toddler is in the habit of creeping into your room during the night and sneaking into your bed while you are asleep, you will need to devise a way of ensuring you wake up before she can get to your room, so you can implement the back-to-bed process and reassurances before she has a chance to get under the covers with you. Keeping the monitor on a loud volume-setting, or blocking your door from the inside so it makes a noise when she tries to open it, are examples of how you can hear her before she arrives!

Although all children respond to sleep-training with a degree of 'individuality', thankfully the majority will respond well. After their initial protests, they will happily accept the changes and the previous sleep issues soon become a distant memory. However, there are a few children who seem more resistant to the changes and protest for a longer period of time, which of course can prove challenging. Perseverance and consistency are key, and as long as you see some positive improvements each night, keep implementing the technique even if it takes two or three weeks.

However, if there is zero or little positive progress, you will need to reassess the situation by checking through all the possible underlying causes of sleep disturbances as listed on p. 91 and referring to Chapter 7 as, if a child doesn't respond to sleep-training, it's very often due to an underlying digestive discomfort.

ALISON SAYS . . .

'I met one little boy who, although he accepted staying in his room, simply refused to sleep in his bed. After we put him to bed he would just get out and curl up on the floor and go to sleep there. The first evening that we watched him do this was quite upsetting, and once he was asleep we went into his room, picked him up and put him on the bed, where he stayed for an hour. He then woke, didn't cry at all, but got out of bed, curled up on the floor again and went back to sleep! We repeated the process of putting him back to bed, but again he woke soon afterwards and went back to his position on the floor. So we decided to leave him there and just went in and covered him with a blanket. In the morning he seemed quite happy and had actually had more sleep in one night than he had ever had before – albeit on the floor!

The next night, in preparation for a repeat performance, we put a cushioned rug and a sheepskin in place and made sure he was wearing warmer pyjamas. Sure enough, after 20 minutes of crying, banging on the door (which he couldn't open), and his mum going in a few times to deliver the sleepy-time phrase, he curled up on the sheepskin, went to sleep and stayed there all night without waking once!

The next evening there weren't even any bedtime tears, but as soon as we left the room he went on to his sheepskin and curled up for the night. It would be another twenty-three days before his mum called to tell me that he had woken up in his bed for the first time! He had started off the night on the rug but had at some point taken himself into his bed. From then on, floor-sleeping was a thing of the past and he continued to sleep happily in his bed with no issues, whatsoever.'

MORNING WAKE-UP MANAGEMENT

Whatever happens during your first night of sleep-training, I truly hope it is easier than you might expect! Unfortunately, it is highly likely that you will all still be tired and a tad stressed, but it is important to see things through with a good morning-wake-up process.

If you have put a sleep-clock or similar timer in place, you will have set a morning 'wake up' on the clock, with an alarm for the same time on your watch or phone. As soon as you know the sleep-clock has shown your toddler it is wake-up time, go into the room and immediately refer to the sleep-clock saying, 'Wow, look, the clock is showing us it's morning and we can get up.' Wave at the clock and try to engage her in acknowledging it, even if she's crying. Then just get her up and enjoy lots of cuddles and kisses, but quite quickly carry on as if everything is totally normal. Don't make a big fuss about anything that happened in the night or make much reference to it.

If she did stay in bed and slept through, give a little praise by saying something simple like, 'Very well done, Sarina, you followed the rules and you stayed in bed and slept all night – that's great.' If she got up, whether once or multiple times, you could still say something positive and cheerful like 'I hope you enjoyed having your new cuddle-cushion and sleep-clock, and I'm sure you will get better at staying in bed as you get used to it.'

SLEEP-TRAINING FOR DAYTIME NAPS

If your child is still requiring a daytime nap but is resistant to going to bed or to sleep, you will need to implement the same reassurance sleep-training technique, with a few adjustments to accommodate the fact that it is nap-time and not night-time.

Use the same sleepy-time phrases and techniques that you use at night for laying your toddler down in the cot or getting them to go back to bed. You can still give the comforters they use for night-time, such as their cuddle-cushion or bunny, but once you've introduced the bedtime rules at night, it's not usually necessary to read these out again for nap-time. If you use white noise then turn this on and, although even with blackout blinds drawn the room will not be pitch black, if they is used to a comforting glow from a night-light then you can turn this on too. If you're using a sleep-clock, use the nap-time setting if you feel it's appropriate.

A successful routine can be trickier to establish at nap-time than at bedtime, and can take longer to be fully accepted by your little one. So many parents find themselves having to lie down with their toddlers during the day as well as at night-time, as it seems to be the only way to get them to nap! Once you've removed the contact-sleep for night-time, you must remove it from the daytime sleep too as it's too confusing for a toddler if you still sleep with them during the day but not at night!

If your toddler only ever naps in a pram for his daytime sleep, you may decide to leave his sleeping in the pram for a few days longer while you focus on getting the nights sorted, then tackle the daytime nap when night sleep is fully established.

EARLY-MORNING WAKING

Many parents are convinced that their toddler was born to be an early riser and are adamant that a 5am wake-up is hard-wired into their child. I have never agreed with this ethos, however, and always believe there is room for improvement!

As mentioned in earlier chapters, while there is variation in individuals' sleep requirements, I will never accept that 5am is the natural wake-up time for any child, and in my opinion the absolute earliest to even think about starting your day would be 6am. Of course, there are exceptions to this rule, and for those parents who do shift work or need to get to the office early in the morning, a very early wake-up for the household may be necessary. Importantly, though, if your toddler is waking before the more natural morning time of 7am, they may not be getting the required sleep quota and sleep deprivation could begin to build.

It is a well-known fact that our biological clocks work on a day–night split, and many sleep scientists suggest that babies and children work on a straight 12-hour divide of each 24-hour period. The Pediatric Sleep Council advises that a natural bedtime for most infants, toddlers and young children is during the early evening, between 6pm and 8pm, and therefore the natural wake-up time in the morning is 12 hours later, between 6am and 8am, so for simplicity I always suggest timings of 7pm to 7am.

Dr Sarah Honaker, who wrote the article for the Pediatric Sleep Council, also alludes to the fact that children are happiest if they are able to wake spontaneously in the morning, without being unnaturally woken – by another person or an alarm, for example. As sleep gets established, you should be able to determine which wake-up time suits your child best; it is advised to keep that time consistent, to within the nearest 30 minutes or less.

Let's look at the main reasons toddlers tend to wake up too early:

- Any milk feeds during the night, whether breast or bottle, will almost certainly be the cause of an early wake-up, as the digestive system itself has to wake up and digest milk when it should be resting.

- Too much sleep during the day can cause early waking, so adjust the daytime nap schedule accordingly and/or limit the total amount of daytime sleep.

- Going to bed too late can, over time, lead to general sleep deprivation. This will cause night-time sleep to deteriorate, so an earlier bedtime is often appropriate. (NB: I advise a 7pm bedtime – 7.30pm latest – for toddlers and children, right up to the age of five years.)

- An acid-reflux problem or dietary intolerance may lie at the root of consistent early waking. (See Chapter 7 for detailed information about this condition.)

- Sometimes early waking has simply become an ingrained habit, which can make it incredibly difficult to break, but sometimes a change of environment – moving your toddler into a different room or just moving his bedroom furniture around – can be enough to break the cycle.

Nearly all early-morning waking needs the same response as for bedtime refusal and night-time wakings, using your reassurances and sleepy-time phrase.

If your toddler has woken before it is time to get up, leave her to see if she will settle back to sleep. If she's getting out of bed or sitting in the bed or cot and crying, then you need to go in and deliver more of the reassurances you used at bedtime and in the night. Once you decide you are going to start your day, you need to go into her room with a bright and cheerful 'Good morning!' Try to ignore the fact that she has been crying; you could say something like 'Why on earth are you making that noise? There's no need to cry; it's time to get up and start our fun day.' If you go in and over-sympathize with her, this will make her feel more upset as she will soak up your recognition of her distress, which then validates it. Of course you are going to want to give her huge cuddles and smother her with love, which is absolutely fine, but shower her with positivity and happiness alongside the love and hugs. Then you can carry on with your normal morning routine as if what happened last night was the most normal thing in the world. Don't let her hear you talking with others about what happened at bedtime or during the night. Just keep a sunny and happy disposition and mentally prepare yourself for nap-time and another bedtime later that day!

Once you've implemented sleep-training, it can take time for the early-morning wake-ups to stop and for your little one's new sleep patterns to fully develop, so try to be patient, be persistent – and persevere. Remember the 'Five Ps' ethos!

A PARENT'S STORY

'My twenty-one-month-old had suffered with awful reflux, and although we got it fully managed, my son always woke early. He would often wake between 4 and 5am, after which he would very rarely go back to sleep. We tried everything, from an earlier bedtime to a later one; more milk at bedtime and no milk. We got him a Groclock, and although he would stay in his cot until the sun-face appeared, he was still awake and would start to call for us, getting louder and louder if we didn't go in. So we used to go in a few times to tell him it was still sleepy-time, before getting him up at 6.45am, when the sun-face came up. The early mornings were killing us. Oddly, the only time our son ever slept through was when we went on holiday to Greece, and he never woke before 7am! We honestly thought that once we got home he would sleep through, having done so for the whole ten nights we were away, but it wasn't to be; our first night back home, he was awake at 4.30am and we were back to normal.

After discussions with Alison, we agreed that he had simply got used to waking early and had learned that, even if we didn't interact with him when we went in to try to settle him, he would get some sort of one-to-one time with us before his older sister got up a bit later. Alison felt he had slept when on holiday because it was a change of environment, so we decided to rearrange the furniture in his room – and amazingly he slept in until 6.30am! To capitalize on this, Alison said that if he woke early again we were to simply leave him until the sun-face came up on his sleep-clock. Sure enough, he woke early again the next morning, so we left him. He was very unhappy and loudly shouted and called for us, but we ignored him. But after waking at 4.15am and protesting until 6, he actually then went back to sleep and we had to wake him up at 7.30! Things gradually improved over the next few mornings and, thankfully, the early waking stopped.'

L. P.

TEARS, CRYING AND TANTRUMS DURING SLEEP-TRAINING

In my first book, *The Sensational Baby Sleep Plan*, I created a 'Crying Scale' to try to help readers decipher the level of their younger baby's cry and whether you need to respond or wait a few more minutes before re-visiting the bedroom to deliver reassurances during sleep-training. Below, I've repeated the baby-focused Crying Scale along with setting a Toddler Tears and Tantrums scale as there is a degree of crossover between the two and it's impossible to pinpoint an exact age when the toddler scale takes over from the baby one – in fact, between twelve and twenty-four months they can both be useful for reference.

The Baby Crying Scale
1. A little whimper: she may grunt and groan on and off for some time, but will not need any reassurance.
2. A small moan: she may whinge and moan a little but will rarely need a visit at this level.
3. An annoyed squawk: she may be getting a little more vocal at this point and just slightly crying, but it is still best to leave her to see whether the cry develops or subsides.

The Baby Crying Scale
4. A frustrated squeal: she may be crying on and off for a few minutes, but with no real conviction and you can actually tell that it is fairly half-hearted.
5. A demanding shout: she may well be loudly vocalizing her displeasure at the turn of events and be missing her dummy, for example, but the cry is not entirely continuous.
6. An escalating cry: she may now be working up to the point where she will not resettle herself and you will need to judge whether or not it is appropriate to go in and give reassurance.
7. A panicky distress call: your baby may sound quite distressed and be crying with only a few brief pauses for breath. If you have not been in for a while, now would definitely be a good time to do so.
8. A very angry yell: a baby can sustain crying at this level for some time, but it is usually out of frustration and anger that things have changed and she doesn't understand why. If you carry out repeated 'sleepy-time' reassurances she will begin to calm down.
9. A full-blown cry: if a true full-on cry does not subside after several minutes, you may need to try another tactic and do a quick reassuring pick-up then put her back down while delivering the sleepy-time message.
10. A blood-curdling scream: using my technique no baby ever reaches this point, as she has already been reassured. I give the number 10 scenario merely to emphasize this scale!
If you find your baby often reaches excessive levels of crying and things don't calm down, see the last chapters of this book and my previous one, The Sensational Baby Sleep Plan, so you can ensure there are no underlying digestive issues causing the distress.

With older toddlers and children, it is much trickier to distinguish a level of cry that merits your attention from one you can leave for a while. This is simply because your baby has grown, as has his lung capacity and his ability to be 'quite loud' with his protests! That said, if you remember how your toddler's brain develops rapidly but still lacks control over emotional responses, it's no wonder they can react with intense crying when you change things. Also, the level of these screaming fits and tantrums will vary from child to child, so it is very difficult to give you an exact guide to follow, but the table below should help you to assess your toddler's level of upset or distress and work out how to respond.

Toddler Tears and Tantrums	
Level of tears	Your response
1. a few sniffles, a couple of moans and a small cry	no visit or reassurances necessary
2. persistent whingeing and calling out	a firm reassurance spoken through the monitor or closed door
3. some intermittent crying and shouts of protest	a quick visit to the room to deliver the reassurance phrase
4. angry shouting and repeated calling out through lots of tears	a few more visits with reassurances, then leaving a longer gap before returning again
5. substantial sobbing, lots of shouting and angry protests	intermittent visits, with a quick mop-up of tears, and delivery of phrase through the monitor or closed door
6. serious crying, wails of despair and calls for help	a visit to the room for a minute or two, repeatedly giving the reassurance phrase, then leaving but repeating a few minutes later if needed

Toddler Tears and Tantrums	
Level of tears	Your response
7. intermittent screaming, crying, sobbing and angry demands	as for previous level but you might stand in the room for longer – perhaps 5 minutes each visit – but without interacting other than to give reassurances
8. very angry shouting and screaming	perhaps standing by the open door so your child can see you, but with minimal interaction or conversation
9. intense screaming, copious tears, any form of self-harm	entering, holding your child firmly in your arms and sitting quietly until he is calm, putting him back to bed and reverting to some of the previous points if he cries again
10. blood-curdling screams, tantrums and even a vomit in protest	perhaps sitting on his bed or a chair, holding him if necessary (and obviously clearing up any vomit) and staying in the room until he is calm before leaving

Although your toddler may reach fever pitch with her responses in the first day or so, it should be fairly short-lived, and if you've implemented everything I have advised then her reactions to the sleep-training should calm down within a few days.

Some children, when in floods of tears, will produce copious amounts of mucus and snot that you may need to wipe away with a damp cloth or hanky each time you go in to deliver a reassurance. I know you will worry about her reacting in this way, and it's definitely upsetting to see, but producing mucus is – if unpleasant – a natural by-product of crying.

One of the worst things to manage when implementing

sleep-training is your toddler vomiting – not through being unwell, but due to excessive crying. If your toddler does vomit due to crying, you'll find it incredibly distressing and feel like the worst parent in the world. In most instances, the children who can easily vomit when they get upset are those who have previously suffered – or still do – from some degree of acid-reflux and/or dietary intolerances. As I always explain, it's vital that any existing issues related to these conditions are fully managed before you embark on sleep-training. However, it is still possible for a child whose condition is managed to vomit due to the crying alone. If this does happen, change all the soiled cot sheets, sleeping bag and your child's night clothes with the minimum of fuss; if possible, try not to even take her out of the cot or bed, and carry out the clean-up process as calmly as possible, then settle her back down and use your sleepy-time reassurances. If you think your toddler is at all likely to vomit, prepare a pile of clean bedding and spare pyjamas prior to bedtime so it will be close to hand.

A PARENT'S STORY

'Our eighteen-month-old hated his cot. Every time we put him in there to sleep, he would literally stand there, cry for a few minutes, then cough and vomit. It was almost as if he had learned to vomit on demand, and he even started doing it in the day if he didn't want to do something! I thought there was something seriously wrong with him, but no medical professional could ever give me an answer; I was just told it was a learned behaviour he would "probably" grow out of. But managing life with our toddler while maintaining some sense of normality for his older brother was almost impossible. Our toddler didn't resist just his cot;

he wouldn't sleep with us either, so we resorted to taking shifts and pushing him in his buggy around the house all night as it was the only way he would sleep! He wouldn't eat solid food, either; just soft, melt-in-the-mouth wafers or crisps, chocolate, yoghurt and certain fruits, but he would never eat a proper meal and I was convinced he couldn't swallow properly. Alison suggested he had acid-reflux and a cow's-milk-protein allergy, and this was confirmed by a paediatric gastroenterologist, who prescribed some medicine and talked us through changing our son's diet. After making all the changes, we saw huge improvements in him, but he would still vomit when protesting, especially if we tried to put him into his cot.

Alison came to stay, and on the first night we did the bath- and bedtime routine with both boys then Alison took our toddler to his room, read him a story and put him in his cot. Sure enough, within minutes he had vomited everywhere, so she went in, changed him and all of the bedding without even picking him up or taking him out of the cot, gave him some water, told him it was 'sleepy-time' and left the room. After 15 minutes more of crying he vomited again, so Alison went in and did exactly the same thing. After another 10 minutes, we watched on the monitor in utter amazement as he simply lay down and just went to sleep! From that night on he accepted going into his cot and never vomited again. He also stopped his daytime "vomit protests" too, and he started to eat proper meals. It took time for this to happen, but the positive change in our little boy was just incredible. Alison simply explained that although we had treated his medical condition, we needed to change his behaviours and learned responses too. Alison is truly a miracle worker and we will be forever in her debt.'

E. S.

If ever you instinctively feel that your toddler really gets *too* upset, is beyond any 'normal' tantrum level or refuses to give in and simply cannot accept the new changes, then I strongly urge you to read the last chapter of this book as it could be that he is just too uncomfortable to lie down and sleep due to an underlying digestive discomfort or dietary intolerance. If this has been ruled out, you can still implement the sleep-training as I've described, but with your own, individual adaptation. For example, after saying goodnight at bedtime, you might decide to sit on the end of the bed, stand in the room or by the door for the first few nights, gradually 'withdrawing' your presence. During this time you might either just stay completely quiet or occasionally deliver your chosen phrase, but remember to use a firm and authoritative tone so your child still understands the difference between awake-time and sleepy-time.

Another method you can use to manage excessive crying by a toddler while sleep-training is 'non-communicative holding'. If you feel your little one is getting too upset and is not calming down, you can go into the room, keeping it as dark as you can, pick up your baby and just hold her. If there's a chair in the room, then you can sit while holding her, but that is *all* you do – hold her. No jigging, rocking, patting, shushing, bouncing, walking around, or singing or talking to her. You almost ignore her; look away, keep a cool, indifferent attitude, and once she calms down say something like, 'Good. You've stopped crying. There is nothing to be crying about and it is still sleepy-time.' As you say this, put her back in the cot and leave the room, repeating the process whenever you feel necessary. Do not allow her to fall asleep in your arms, as that will defeat the whole process; although it's OK if she gets sleepy, she does need to be aware that you are putting her back to bed.

☆ ALISON'S GOLDEN RULES ☆

1. Ensure that your toddler is well and not suffering from any degree of digestive discomfort before implementing sleep-training.

2. Remember to use the ethos of the 'Five Ps': plan, prepare, patience, persistence and perseverance.

3. Clear your diary for a week or more after you begin sleep-training.

4. Remember to adopt an attitude in line with the 'Five Cs': calm, controlled, confident, clear, consistent.

5. Devise your sleepy-time phrase and use it throughout sleep-training and beyond. Make sure the other people involved with your baby's sleep-times use exactly the same phrase.

6. Enlist as much help as possible from family members or friends, even if they just come round to offer moral support.

7. Ensure that everyone involved in the care of your toddler understands the technique and how to use it, displaying unity from all adult caregivers.

8. Remember to read and refer to the new bedtime rules you created with your toddler as part of the bedtime routine.

9. Try to remain aloof and indifferent when delivering your sleepy-time reassurances and not to respond to all your toddler's demands or questions.

10. Once your toddler is asleep in her own bed and in her own room for the first time ever, go ahead and celebrate with a glass or two – but be prepared for further night-time wakings!

CHAPTER 6

Siblings, Travel and the Toilet

You now know exactly how to implement the changes necessary to enable your toddler to look forward to bedtime, to fall asleep independently and happily enjoy a full night's sleep. Once everything has settled down and adequate sleep has been restored, you can enjoy calm and pleasant evenings while your toddler is safely tucked up in bed – but beware the false sense of security! All too quickly there will be changes ahead that can throw the proverbial spanner in the works and test you with yet more night-time challenges!

The following factors, in particular, are likely to affect your toddler's sleep routine, but I have tips and advice to help you manage all of them.

THE SIBLING DYNAMIC

The best preparation for the arrival of a new baby is to ensure your firstborn is happily sleeping in his own bed, in his own room, right through the night, with a set bath- and bedtime routine beforehand. Being well-rested and feeling secure within his daily routine will help your toddler feel less challenged by the arrival of a new sibling.

It is very exciting for a toddler when a new baby arrives, but it may sometimes have a negative impact on her sleep as she may be disturbed by the baby's cries and hear you during the night as you are up giving night-time feeds, while also experiencing mounting feelings of jealousy when she realizes that baby is sleeping in your room! Whether or not your toddler used to sleep in with you, it's understandable that a new baby sleeping in your room can make your toddler feel left out.

You can of course try to explain that when babies are very new, they have to sleep next to Mummy, just as your toddler did when she was a little baby. Show your toddler all her baby photos and dress your baby in some of the clothes you have kept, telling your toddler that she used to wear the same outfits when she was a baby. Also explain that when your little one was a baby, she too slept in Mummy's room and, as the new baby gets older, he will move into his own room just as your toddler has done.

However, no matter what reactions there are from your toddler, it is always best to try not to overcompensate or to allow any leeway with your toddler's behaviour, especially when it comes to bedtime and sleep. Typically – and often through your own feelings of guilt at having disrupted your toddler's life – you may feel compelled to relax the rules and, for example, stay longer with your toddler at bedtime or let her sleep in your room for a night or two so she doesn't feel left out, but this is a slippery slope, and before you know it all the positive sleep associations you have previously established could disappear, and you will then have to manage an overtired, overemotional toddler as well as your new baby. Your toddler will actually feel more reassured and secure if her usual routine and boundaries remain firmly in place, as opposed to experiencing feelings of uncertainty that can build as you suddenly allow her to do things that were previously not acceptable.

There has to be some acceptance that life has changed and that the new baby is here to stay. That said, wherever possible try to keep your toddler's usual routine in place. That might mean asking someone else to do the nursery run or perhaps to watch the baby for a short while so you can take your toddler to nursery, enjoying some brief one-to-one time on the way. In fact, any one-to-one attention will be felt as a huge positive by your toddler, so if a friend or family member can spare an hour to come over to play with her, it will boost her self-esteem.

ALISON SAYS . . .

'Whether it's the arrival of a new baby, moving home, a family loss or even enduring months of lockdown due to a pandemic, in all stressful and challenging situations the one thing to try to keep consistent is for your babies, toddlers and children to happily accept bedtime each evening and continue to sleep through the night. Not only do you then have evenings free to breathe and relax a little, but when your children are properly rested they are much easier to manage during the day than if they are sleep-deprived.'

Many parents want to share the news with their toddler as soon as they find out they're pregnant, but I advise to wait if you can. Toddlers can really only understand things that are tangible – things that they can see, hold, examine and touch. They struggle to understand the concept of something without a physical presence or image, as their brain has simply not reached that level of maturity. You can give them a pretend 'baby' or doll, along with all the accessories like nappies, clothing and a pushchair, and try to explain that Mummy is soon going to have a new baby to look after too, but your toddler will not really be able to relate the doll to the reality of a new baby arriving. Similarly, your toddler will find it difficult to understand 'going on holiday' as she simply can't visualize the place you will be visiting. You can show her pictures or even videos of where you're going, but she still won't have any understanding of what the 'holiday' will entail.

With this in mind, seven or eight months is a long time for them to be hearing talk of a new brother or sister arriving when they can't understand the concept. Obviously, you may have friends who have already had a new baby and your toddler's playmates will have become older brothers or sisters who you can refer to as examples, but she still won't understand how her own life will change and what impact the new arrival may have on the family as a whole. So, my advice is to wait until your bump really starts to show, at around six months. This still gives you time to make any physical changes you may need to make to your home environment. For example, you may decide to transition your toddler to a bed so that the cot is free for when baby needs it, and although that's unlikely to be for some months, it is far better to make the transition sooner rather than later. This means your toddler will not make the connection that things are changing 'because of the baby', which can easily allow feelings of resentment to build. Similarly, if you're going to need to move your toddler from one bedroom to another, then do it before she knows about the baby's impending arrival and therefore without her knowing that the change is happening because baby will need what was her room!

My general rule of thumb in these situations is to either make the changes around three months before baby arrives or, if this isn't possible, not until baby is at least three months old. In the latter case, your toddler has plenty of time before and after the baby's arrival to adjust to the new situation without feeling that she has had to give things up or that the physical changes in the house are made solely in honour of the baby.

Here is a common scenario and my advice on how to proceed:

You are six months into your pregnancy and your toddler is twenty months old. She is still in a cot in the smaller bedroom, which is closest to yours. There is a toddler bed in the larger bedroom that you want to move her into; the baby will have the cot in the smaller room once you move the infant out of your room.

Remembering my advice about transitioning from cot to bed between eighteen and twenty-four months, you could make the change right away without your toddler realizing that the move is really being made because of the new baby. Then, when you move the baby out of your room and into the cot in the smaller room, your toddler will almost have forgotten she used to sleep in there and will have been happily settled in her bed in the larger room for a number of months. She will therefore have little reason to feel jealous or that she has been usurped by her younger sibling!

Or you might decide to wait and make the changes after the baby has arrived, which is also fine as long as you approach the situation with care. Once your baby has reached three or four months, you may want to move him out of your room and put him in the cot in the small bedroom. (NB: The NHS guidelines state that a baby should sleep in your room until six months of age, but many parents choose to move their baby out sooner than this. If you decide to move him at this earlier time, put an under-mattress sensor in place to make sure he is completely safe, and for peace of mind.) This means also moving your now twenty-seven-month-old toddler to the new room and into a bed.

Hopefully, you've followed my first book, *The Sensational Baby Sleep Plan*, and your baby is already sleeping through the night, so the move into the big cot should be quite easy, with little disruption to the baby's sleep. By following all the advice detailed in the first five chapters of this new book, your first-born's transition into the new room and toddler bed should be just as smooth.

The main thing to remember when approaching the change is to ensure your older child doesn't feel the change is being made because the baby now needs her cot, but rather that she is simply getting too big for the cot and needs a bed. During the week or so prior to making the move, you could host bedtime stories on the bed in the bigger room, which will help get your toddler used to being in the room. On the day you decide to make the change, let her have the usual daytime nap or quiet-time in the cot, then use the afternoon to move her things to her new room, create the bedtime rules and put her name on the door.

I would suggest you leave the old room empty for a week or two before moving your baby into the cot, as this will give your toddler time to adjust and it won't be so obvious to her that the move was instigated by her younger sibling's need for her cot. In fact, as soon as your toddler seems settled in her new room, you could 'pretend' to her that you have an idea and exclaim, 'It would be a really great idea to move the baby out of our room now and into the empty cot, so everyone has their own room.'

Of course, you could choose to make the move for both your

toddler and baby at the same time, but you must still make sure your toddler believes the reason for the move is because she needs a bigger bed to sleep in, and that moving the baby into the cot is almost just an afterthought.

When baby arrives home

Aside from the physical changes in your home to accommodate a new baby, there will also be emotional ones to contend with, especially for your older child or children. Interestingly, I have found that the older your child before a new baby arrives, the less they seem disturbed or unsettled by the new arrival. A five-year-old, for example, will likely be at school during the day and have a fairly structured social life, with friends to see, as well as clubs and classes a few times a week, whereas a younger toddler may be home more of the time, will see you spending lots of time with the new baby and is not as emotionally mature. For them, this can easily result in an outpouring of feelings such as anger, jealousy, upset, aggression and frustration, which can be quite upsetting for everyone.

Despite any preparation you may have put in place, and all the explanations you've provided for your toddler about the imminent arrival of a new baby, nothing can truly prepare her. In the blink of an eye, not only has this new, crying 'thing' turned up, but Mummy also disappeared for a night or two, which may not have happened before, and it can actually be the latter that upsets your toddler more than the new baby arriving.

In preparation, and to help your toddler to better cope with the likelihood of Mummy going to hospital when the baby comes, try to get her used to other people helping with, or actually 'doing' bedtime, so she is not completely reliant on one particular person putting her to bed each evening. If possible, arrange for your toddler to go and stay overnight with grandparents or another close family member, so she gets used to staying with other people, and when the time comes for the baby to arrive, your toddler can be safely and happily looked after, away from all the excitement, stress and drama that might surround labour and the birth.

Of course, you would never want to exclude your toddler completely, and she needs to be involved to some degree with the arrival of her new sibling, but for the most part she will generally feel more settled by being somewhat shielded.

ALISON SAYS . . .

'Years ago, children going to stay with grandparents, for example, was a much more common occurrence than it is today. This is partly due to the fact that many of us move away from family, even to different countries, but it's also because of recent "perfect parenting" pressures that seem to suggest you're a bad parent if you send your child to stay with others; that to be the "best Mummy" you literally have to do it all yourself! Also, many years ago the usual length of a hospital stay after having a baby was a minimum of four or five days, and typically grandparents or other family members would look after the older children while Mum and baby stayed in hospital. This allowed time for everyone to get used to the new situation, with the older children visiting Mummy and the new baby in hospital. Sadly, the situation today is vastly different and it feels like there is often much more panic and stress surrounding the imminent birth, as women, once in labour, have to remain at home longer before going to hospital and are often discharged within 24 hours of giving birth, arriving home completely exhausted. It can be such a fraught few days, from the onset of labour, rushing to hospital and then arriving back home with the new baby, and many toddlers and older children can be rather traumatized by the emotionally charged chain of events, with little time to adjust or to process what's actually happening.'

PARENTAL GUILT

The physical changes that need to be made in your home to accommodate your new baby are, in all honesty, much easier to manage than the emotional changes you will experience as your family expands, and none more so than maternal guilt. As parents with a newborn and toddler sibling – and this goes for mothers, especially – we tend to pile the guilt on ourselves and worry about everything, such as:

- turning your firstborn's life upside down
- not having enough time to bond with your new baby
- not having enough time to spend with your toddler
- that your toddler is now being entertained by the 'virtual babysitter'
- leaving your baby to cry for a few minutes while you cook a meal and feed your toddler
- not being able to replicate for your new baby the same time and attention you gave your toddler when they were born

- worrying about your seemingly deteriorating relationship with your partner

- feelings of guilt that you don't seem to be coping with looking after two children and that you need help

- feeling guilty that you almost wish you hadn't decided to have another baby

- feeling that you're not meeting anybody's needs

- feeling frustrated and not even finding the time to shower, let alone go to the loo in peace

- even when your children are sleeping, not being able to get to sleep yourself as you're so anxious that one or both of them will wake, and that this lack of sleep will make you even more tired the next day and even less able to cope

- feeding guilt: whether it's because breastfeeding is taking too much time away from your toddler or because you're not breastfeeding as you can't find the time to make it work

Many fathers experience feeling varying degrees of guilt linked to not feeling 'useful' enough, still having to go to work and not being at home to help more.

Most second- and third-time parents will identify with many of the above points, which I find sad in so many ways. My ethos is simply to try to celebrate your successes and don't worry so much about the things that don't seem to come together. All your children will thrive and survive, but, if it makes you feel better, start a savings account called 'Kids' Therapy Fund', which they can access when they're older – it's highly likely they won't really need it, and then you can use the funds to reward yourself with a well-deserved treat for being such an awesome and amazing parent!

MANAGING BEDTIME WITH MORE THAN ONE CHILD

Once a new baby arrives, one of the most challenging scenarios is bath- and bedtime. How on earth do you manage to keep your toddler's usual evening routine from being disrupted while also meeting the needs of your baby, who wants to cluster-feed and is at her most unsettled at this time of day? The answer: quite simply, you can't! Or perhaps you can – if you are able to accept in your mind that your toddler's life has changed and things will simply never be the same as they were before the new baby arrived.

The sooner you can acknowledge, without any guilt, that there is a new member of the family to look after and that life is going to be very different, the sooner your toddler will get used to the changes too. The best advice for managing bath- and bedtime with one or more older children and a new baby is to ask for help. Beg or plead for help at the children's bedtime from whoever you can, as it's likely to be the most challenging time of day until your new baby is at least six or eight weeks old, so an extra pair of hands will be hugely helpful!

It can be interesting to recall how you created the most wonderfully calm and happy bedtime routine with your eldest child, but can only provide a somewhat 'watered-down' version for each subsequent child, which shows how much children's birth order has an effect on how they grow up. That said, whether you are trying to manage solo or do have help, the following list will give you plenty of tips to help make bedtime easier:

- Rather than trying to stagger the children's bathtimes, try to combine them from the start. Even if you have a four-year-old and a new baby, I would still try to do bathtime with them both at the same time, then afterwards your older child can relax with some books or an audio-story while you feed your baby and then settle her to bed. If your child shows an interest, get him to 'help' wash, dry or dress the new baby, which will make your child feel included and important.

- Sometimes you might bath your baby on her own, but with your toddler 'helping'. Then, while you feed baby – perhaps sitting on the loo seat – your older child has his bath, but still with lots of supervision and vocal interaction from you.

- Remembering the advice to limit screen time for a couple of hours before bed, you could leave your older child listening to an audiobook in his room or on your bed while you feed your baby then settle her to bed. You then do a quicker version of bath- and bedtime with your toddler, but at least it is still on a one-to-one basis.

- It might prove easier to make your baby's schedule slightly later than that of your toddler. For example, if your toddler is used to having a bath at 6pm and being asleep by 7pm each evening, you could try to give your baby a late-afternoon feed around 5pm or even 6pm, and then let the baby sleep while you bathe your toddler then put him to bed. Of course, you then have to do another bath- and bedtime with your baby, which can make for a long evening!

- It's quite possible that, previously, your toddler was very easy to put to bed and happily settled himself to sleep, but since the arrival of your new baby he has suddenly become quite challenging and refusing to go to bed. This is a natural reaction and likely caused by jealousy, but it is important to try to keep the usual routine in place and stick to the sleep-training, as opposed to overcompensating by relaxing the usual bedtime rules.

- There may be times when your toddler has to take a back seat and allow you uninterrupted time to see to your new baby. This will be difficult for your toddler to accept, but also a good life lesson, which will ultimately help him to learn that we are all equal and that his new sibling is as important as he is.

- If you are too tired, the day has not gone to plan and you simply can't face doing bathtime with any of your little ones, then just bypass it! Instead, engineer a quick wash of hands and faces, and clean some teeth, then get everyone changed into pyjamas and snuggling on your bed for an audio-story, saving you having to read, with milk feeds for those that need them and winding-down-time all round.

SLEEP-TRAINING MORE THAN ONE CHILD AT A TIME

There are so many different elements to consider when you have more than one child to manage throughout the night, and so many different set-ups. For example, you may have:

- your baby and toddler in separate rooms

- your baby and toddler sharing a room

- twins or triplets sharing a room

- twins in separate rooms

- a four-year-old and a two-year-old who now need to share as your new baby needs to go into his own room

- three or more children, all in separate rooms

Whatever your individual situation when it comes to how many children you have, their ages and the available beds and bedroom space you have, my sleep-training technique will still work.

Parents are often worried that their one non-sleeping baby or toddler will disturb their other child, who may be a great sleeper, and this easily leads to bad habits forming, with parents reacting too quickly and doing anything possible to keep their wakeful child quiet and get them back to sleep. Whether that means giving a bottle of milk, a breastfeed, rocking them back to sleep or even taking them into your bed, anything seems preferable to their sleeping child or children being woken, as they would then have two or more wakeful children to manage.

At some point, however, the decision may be made to improve the situation and implement reassurance sleep-training. Though you might, understandably, be concerned about disturbing your child who does sleep well, most parents are surprised how little the noise made by one child at night will actually disturb the other. For example, I've worked with many twins and triplets over the years, and in most cases they've all shared a bedroom – yet whether it was one triplet who didn't sleep well, both twins or just one of them who needed sleep-training, the children who did sleep were rarely disturbed by the cries of their siblings.

Quite simply, whether your children are all in the same room or all sleeping separately, you will need to apply my sleep-training technique, as described in Chapter 5, to all of them at once – even the good sleeper – and treat them all the same. More often than not, siblings will not disturb each other at night, but obviously it can happen and I appreciate you may feel sorry for your good sleeper, who may be disturbed during the first night or two and get woken up by the cries of your other child. However, rather than giving in to your emotions, overcompensating and trying to comfort her, just deliver your sleepy-time reassurance phrases and soon enough she'll very likely go back to sleep.

If you have two or more crying children in different rooms, then visit each room in turn to deliver your reassurances. Remember to be consistent and say the same phrase to each child, as they will feel more reassured if they are all being treated in exactly the same way.

For example, you may have a seven-month-old baby, a twenty-two-month-old toddler and a four-year-old, all in different rooms, and it is only the toddler who doesn't sleep well. Nonetheless, to ensure the other children don't feel left out, it might be an idea to put all three names at the top of your bedtime rules, allow all three children to contribute to the decoration of the poster and place it in a more communal place, near all the bedrooms – on the landing, for example. Alternatively, you could let them each create a different poster for themselves. Similarly, though your older child doesn't *need* a sleep-clock, for example, putting one in place for him anyway will prevent any feelings of jealousy; and whatever comforter you may decide to put in place for the toddler, it's a good idea to also get one for your older child and even the baby. Obviously, due to safety guidelines, you need to be mindful of putting comforters in place for your baby, so if, for example, you get a photo-printed cushion for the older two, maybe you could get the same photo imposed on the sheet that the baby sleeps on to ensure they are all treated as equally as possible. Otherwise, your good sleepers will witness your toddler being rewarded with loads of one-to-one attention, getting to decorate the rules and being given a special clock or a 'Mummy pillow', for example – all because she isn't sleeping at night!

ALISON SAYS . . .

'I was asked to help a family who had a three-and-a-half-year-old boy and a seven-month-old baby. The parents had co-slept with the toddler for some time since he was a baby, and had managed to get him into his own room only with one of them sleeping on a mattress on the floor next to his cot until he went to sleep. Then, every time he woke, one of them would have to go back in and lie down again until the child went back to sleep.

The parents hadn't set out to co-sleep or take turns on a mattress in their toddler's room, but they had never been successful with any kind of sleep-training. It had taken them so long to get any help to manage the child's severe reflux and cow's-milk allergy that by the time he was eighteen months, and even though most of the symptoms were under control, his negative sleep associations had become deeply ingrained. He was in so much discomfort because of his reflux and cow's-milk allergy that he had never been able to sleep and he was therefore almost fearful of bedtime, knowing that it would lead to a very uncomfortable night. It had become a hugely stressful situation and Mum and Dad just didn't know how to change things.

Once the baby had arrived, the toddler's sleep got worse, with more wake-ups, resulting in Dad sleeping on the floor mattress for the whole night. Meanwhile, Mum was co-sleeping with the baby, who unbeknown to his parents also had severe reflux and cow's-milk allergy. The baby had never napped in his cot, only in the sling or pram, and was woken for multiple feeds in the night.

After a few phone calls with me, and following my

advice, they saw a doctor who prescribed acid-reducing omeprazole and a special milk for the baby. I then went to stay with the family and put the baby's cot into his brother's room, as they needed to share a bedroom due to limited space in the house.

I managed to get the baby to sleep for 45 minutes in his cot during the first afternoon, which was a huge achievement. I also created some "bedtime rules" and encouraged the three-year-old to help me decorate them with stickers. The rules were put up on the wall in the boys' bedroom, to be read out each night as part of the bedtime routine. So, after bath, milk, stories, and goodnight kisses and cuddles, both boys went into their cots, then it was lights out, door closed and a firm "It's sleepy-time now" message.

There were tears of protest from both, and the three-year-old shouted for Dad numerous times, but, after a few reassurances, just 10 minutes later they had both calmed down and were sleeping! The older boy woke again after 45 minutes and cried for another 25 minutes, but, again, with a few reassurances he was soon back to sleep.

The baby woke at 2am and 6am, crying on and off for 20 minutes each time, but he quite easily re-settled and both boys slept until 7.30am! The fascinating fact to note here is that each time one of the boys woke and cried, the noise *didn't* wake the other one up. This isn't a surprise to me but the parents were in shock!

The next night, I switched the older boy's cot for a proper bed and put the baby into the larger cot with the sides in place. There was little protest at bedtime:

the baby went straight to sleep and the toddler only got out of bed once before settling to sleep – and they both slept through the whole night without *any* wake-ups. They continued to sleep well from that night on, and the family's sleep was restored.'

ILLNESS AND TEETHING

Though you will have made absolutely certain your toddler is fit and well before instigating sleep-training, once she is sleeping through the night and readily taking her daytime naps, be aware that any new illness or the discomfort of teething may cause her to wake again during the night. Obviously you will need to look after her and administer medicine, water, comfort and cuddles along with whatever else may be required, but ideally it is best to do this while keeping her in her own room and otherwise continuing with the routine. You will unravel everything you've achieved up to now if you give back all the sleep associations and sleep-crutches you've removed, and this would also be very confusing for your toddler.

That said, it is highly possible you may need to manage things in a different way while she is unwell and resort to sleeping with her in her room, taking her to a different room to sleep or even taking her into your bed. Once she is well, you can revert back to using your reassurances and sleep-training technique to re-instil a full night's sleep and eradicate any bad habits that may have developed or recurred while she was unwell.

THE UK SEASONAL HOUR-CHANGE

Just as you've implemented the sleep-training, your little ones are sleeping and, for the first time in months, you start getting a full night's sleep, the clocks change and throw the proverbial spanner in the works.

When the hour goes forward or back, in autumn and spring respectively, it can be quite a challenging time for some parents, who worry how they are going to get their little ones to adapt. However, over the years many parents have told me that, oddly, the hour-change seemed to help create a better sleep pattern and their children actually slept better! I'm certain that this is more true of the hour-change in the autumn, as children's natural sleep patterns and body clock seem to be better suited to the darker evenings.

Once your child is properly sleeping through the night, it is fairly easy to alter his body clock by extending or shortening his 12-hour day or 12-hour night. His biological clock is already naturally programmed to understand the difference between night and day and you can adjust his bedtime and wake-up time to fall in line when the hour-change occurs.

There are a number of ways to adapt to the hour-change. For example:

- Since the hour-change always occurs in the early hours of a Sunday, when you hopefully have no early commitments, you could just get up with your child at the normal wake-up time (yesterday's 7am, for example) and reset things by implementing the usual hour for bedtime (the new 7pm but yesterday's 6 or 8pm).

- If you use a sleep-clock, you could reset the wake-up time by daily increments of 15 or 30 minutes from the day of the hour-change, to gradually 'soak up' the hour difference.

- If it's about to be the spring hour-change, when the clocks go forward and we lose an hour, reaching bedtime sooner, you might decide to use this opportunity to stop daytime naps and do bedtime an hour earlier than normal, in the hope that your toddler still goes to sleep easily and enjoys a longer night-time sleep.

- When the clocks go back again, in the autumn, we gain an extra hour in the night – but of course your toddler doesn't know this, so he will likely wake at the new 6am, as to him it's still 7am. To manage this, leave your child in bed for as long as you can in the morning, even if he's awake, then get him up at the new 7am and carry on with your normal daily schedule. Serving meals at the newly adjusted times can be a massive help, and within a matter of days his body clock should have fairly easily aligned itself and accepted the new time.

- You might find it easier to adapt the hour-change by altering the time of bath- and bedtime and putting your child to bed either slightly earlier or later, depending on which way the hour is changing.

You may decide to synchronize the hour-change with implementing the reassurance sleep-training technique as it can be beneficial to get it all over in one go, rather than establishing a sleep pattern in your toddler that you then have to alter only a few days later.

Changing time-zones

Travelling can be challenging at the best of times when you have little ones, but even more so when going abroad and travelling to a different time-zone. The dilemma of whether or not to travel overseas with your little ones and risk upsetting their sleep patterns is one many parents have to face, and the advice surrounding the issue is varied, to say the least! Some say: 'Do all your travelling while they are still babes in arms and before they reach the toddler stage, as they'll be unaware of what's happening, will stay where you put them and are easier to manage.' Others advise: 'Wait until they are toddlers or older, as they can better appreciate the experience and you can explain the whole travelling scenario to them.'

ALISON SAYS . . .

'I offered some practical tips and advice for travelling with babies in my first book, *The Sensational Baby Sleep Plan*. However, one of the most memorable pieces of advice I've heard about travelling with little ones was imparted by my mother. At the age of seventy-eight, she was helping me to write my first book; her knowledge of grammar, punctuation and good English was invaluable. When I told her I wanted to write about "time-zone travel with your baby", my mother asked what I meant. I explained about the popularity of worldwide travel today and her reply was quick and simple: "How ridiculous, dear – just tell them not to blooming well bother!" We both laughed, and in some respects my mother's words were actually sound advice, but most of us will travel at some point with our children so it helps to have some tips up your sleeve to make the experience easier.'

The simplest way to ensure easy travel and your toddler's quick acceptance of a change in time-zone is to have a well-established bath-, bedtime and night-time sleeping schedule in place before you go, which will also mean that your child's body clock is already programmed to associate meals with daytime, followed by sleep at night. Depending on where you are travelling to, you may need to lengthen the day of travel and shorten that night, or vice versa, and this can be more easily achieved if your child's body clock is already following the natural bio-rhythms of the sun and the moon and is set to understand the difference between day and night.

If you are travelling to a country that is 8 hours behind GMT, for example, you will need to extend the day by keeping your toddler up. Although she will be very tired and need to sleep, once you arrive at your destination aim to fit in with local time as quickly as possible. Of course, she may well fall asleep and this is fine, but don't let her sleep for hours on end – as tempting as this may be! As soon as you can, try to implement as near-normal as possible a bath- and bedtime routine, and properly settle your toddler to bed – but be prepared for some resistance, tears and even tantrums. Most of this upset will be due to overtiredness, and although you may be exhausted yourself and feel like 'doing anything possible' to get your little one to quieten down and go to sleep, remember the sleep-training ethos and use your sleepy-time reassurances until your little one is settled.

It might take a couple of days for your child to fully adjust to the new time-zone, but in general I have found that the outward journey is easier to adapt to and takes less time than the homeward one; as a rough guide, you can expect the outward change to take 24 hours per 2-hour time difference, while on the way back it tends to take 24 hours for each 1-hour difference. This means that for a 6-hour time difference you could expect a three-day adjustment period on the way out and a six-day adjustment period on the way back. Alternatively, if you are travelling to Greece, for example, where there is only a 2-hour time difference, you could decide to keep your toddler's routine within the English time-frame of 7am to 7pm for the duration of your holiday, which in effect means you would do 9am to 9pm Greek time, and I know of many people who have found this to work really well.

Even with the above advice, some people choose to simply go with the flow, eschew any set routine and allow sleep to happen 'as and when' – even perhaps all sleeping in the same bed – and then re-establish the schedule when they get back. It is, of course, up to you, but do remember that it may then take up to a week to get things back on track.

POTTY-TRAINING: THE BASICS

Potty-training comes in two halves: day and night! However, most toddlers will learn to use the potty or toilet during the day long before they are dry at night. This can have a huge effect on bedtime sleep, so it's worth familiarizing yourself with the basics of potty-training before looking at dry nights specifically.

As with most of my advice about managing changes with your little one, I advise you to keep potty-training as simple as possible and not to over-sensationalize the transition out of nappies to using the toilet.

Through my extensive work with babies and children, I have met families from many different cultures and countries, each of whom have different beliefs and follow different traditions when it comes to raising a child – not least when it comes to toilet habits. In many developing-world countries, toilet-training begins almost from birth using an approach now known in the West as the 'elimination-communication' technique, in which babies are taught to urinate and defecate when prompted by a sound made by the parent or carer, and without the use of nappies.

Given our global effort to try to reduce plastic waste, this technique is becoming more popular across the world as many parents attempt to reduce the use of disposable nappies. Others are exploring alternative eco-friendly options, such as washable nappies and biodegradable or recyclable wipes, or those that are made with recycled materials. Be aware, however, that only 50–80 per cent of a so-called biodegradable nappy will actually biodegrade! And should you choose to use washable nappies and opt for cotton cloths instead of disposable wipes, bear in mind how much extra water, washing powder and conditioner this may use.

Signs that your toddler is ready to transition from nappies can be visible from as early as eighteen months, especially if he has an older sibling who leads by example, but he may not show signs of being ready until he is three years old.

The most common signs that your toddler is ready to move out of nappies are:

- He is dry for at least 3 hours at a time and you notice you are having to change fewer nappies.

- He will often wake from a nap with a dry nappy.

- When he wakes in the morning, his nappy is still dry and clean.

- His bowel movements have been regular for some time.

- He protests at nappy-changing.

- He resists putting on a nappy.

- He communicates in some way that he is doing a pee or a poop.

- He is able to pull his own trousers up and down.

- Even though he is still wearing a nappy, he chooses to go and hide when he does a poop – and sometimes for a pee. This indicates that he is completely aware of his bodily functions and knows when he needs to 'go'.

- He gets upset about doing a poop in his nappy and then doesn't like you changing it.

- He vocalizes his desire to use the toilet or sit on the potty.

- He asks to wear pants instead of nappies.

If your child shows three or more of these signs, then it's likely he is ready to transition and my advice is to give it a try.

In an ideal scenario, you would wait until you've got a week where you can stay at home, with no other distractions or commitments, to focus only on making the transition, but life rarely affords us the ideal scenario and you may just have to crack on with it regardless, as soon as your toddler seems ready. There is no prerequisite to use a potty before transitioning to the toilet or that you must use only one or the other. I personally think it's best to look at your home environment and use what works best for you.

Here are some top tips:

- Prepare your toddler by allowing him or her to accompany you to the toilet and explain what's happening. They will quickly realize that going to the loo is quite normal, but will also understand from your demonstration or explanation that girls and boys are different and might perform the act in a different way. Normalizing the use of the toilet from an early age can be hugely beneficial in 'toilet-training' your child.

- Encourage him to help you flush the loo after you have been, so he gets used to seeing the waste being flushed away.

- Talk him through the basic physiology of digestion – that what goes in must come out.

- Let him watch nature programmes where it shows animals having a pee or poop so he can see that all animals need to do it.

- Try to remove any embarrassing stigma and normalize everything about how the human body functions: we all have the same 'equipment' in one form or another!

- If you are going to use a potty, make sure it is sturdy enough and not likely to tip over when your toddler excitedly sits on it or quickly stands up to 'examine' his produce.

- Avoid dressing your toddler in tight-fitting pants or knickers, as the snug fit and elastication around the waist and thighs can make him feel like he's wearing a nappy and make him forget he's wearing pants.

- If possible, don't even use pants for the first day or so of potty-training and let him run free.

- When your toddler has an 'accident', don't berate him; just express your disappointment that he forgot to use the potty or toilet.

- Don't keep asking him every 5 minutes if he needs to pee; it will only irritate him and make him less likely to want to use the toilet.

- When he succeeds in doing a pee or a poop in the potty or the toilet, give some positive praise, but don't go over the top and try to keep it all fairly calm.

Above all, when your toddler says he needs to pee or poop, try not to overreact and think you've got to rush him to the toilet that instant. Toilet-training is not just about teaching a toddler to pee or poop in a toilet, but about them learning to control their bodily functions and 'holding on' for a few minutes between realizing they need to go and actually going. So when your little one tells you he needs to 'go', respond with 'OK, hold on for just a minute, then I can help you,' rather than creating a huge drama about getting him to the loo. Holding on obviously takes time for toddlers to master, and might actually cause a few more accidents in the first few days. However, very quickly your child will learn that they can do it, and in the longer-term this leads to your child understanding that he can control his need for the toilet, by both day and night.

Becoming dry at night

(NB: I haven't mentioned night-time pooping here as all healthy digestive systems will expel the waste come the morning and not through the night. If, while still in nappies or indeed not, your child is pooping at night, she is certainly not ready for toilet-training and I would urge you to read Chapter 7 to explore the possible reasons why she is having bowel movements at night.)

It should be relatively easy to pinpoint when your child is ready to stop wearing nappies at night, as you will find that her nappy is dry when she wakes up after a nap or in the morning and she waits to pee in the toilet instead. A dry nappy on four consecutive mornings is also a sign she is ready. However, she may not ask to go to the toilet and prefer to do her morning pee in her night nappy, so make sure the first thing you do upon wake-up is to remove the nappy and encourage her to use the toilet. All too often I've seen toddlers who are dry throughout the day but then stay and 'use' their night nappy for too long after getting up in the morning, which can then encourage daytime accidents to occur. Your child may also indicate that she is ready to not wear a nappy through the night by protesting at having the nappy put on or even taking it off once she's in bed.

Getting your toddler dry at night might seem like quite a challenge, and it can certainly take time, but it's important that you remain patient – even if you seem to be changing endless wet bed sheets and the washing machine is constantly on! There are no hard and fast rules for how to achieve it, but it may be useful to remember the following:

- Night-time dryness doesn't happen at the same time as daytime training. It can take months or even years for some children to master it, so don't take away bedtime nappies until you feel your toddler is ready.

- Be calm when bed-wetting happens. If your toddler wets the bed, don't tell her off or scold her. Try to change the bed and her nightwear with the minimum of fuss and interaction, staying as calm as possible so you are not inadvertently giving her lots of attention for the 'accident'.

- Provide easy access to a toilet or potty. You could place a particularly sturdy potty or toddler-toilet in her room if there isn't clear or easy access to the family toilet. You will likely need to put a night-light somewhere so she can see what she's doing, and you may need to supervise night-time potty use as it will likely need emptying.

- Encourage your toddler to manage her toilet needs herself during the night and not to be reliant on your input and help.

- Make sure you give loose-fitting nightwear that your toddler can easily manage herself, and help her practise pulling clothes up or down when she needs to use the toilet at night.

- Add a toilet trip to the end of your toddler's bedtime routine. Make the toilet the last stop before bed so your toddler's bladder will be empty before she goes to sleep.

- Use protective sheets, a mattress protector or disposable bed pads under your toddler's top sheet as it will make night-time bed changes much easier. Have clean bedding, towels and clean nightwear close to hand and leave a light on outside your toddler's room, so you can see what you're doing with minimal fuss.

- Consider waking your toddler for a 'dream pee' – lifting your toddler out of bed late in the evening, taking them to the loo, then putting them back to bed. However, some children don't respond to this, either because they are in such a deep sleep and you can't wake them, or because you disturb their sleep and they can't settle back to sleep for ages.

- Don't rush your toddler's night-time dryness. If you have three dry nights in a row things are working, but if there's absolutely no progression after this then you may need to consider putting her back in nappies and trying again in a month's time. It's certainly preferable to broken nights and endless washing. And don't worry – they all get there in the end!

Toilet protests at bedtime

Many toddlers who are resistant to going to bed and settling for the night will use delaying-tactics to drag out the bedtime process, including insisting they need to use the toilet – often multiple times. It amazes me how quickly many of them realize that you will find it hard to ignore their demand to go to the loo!

If you've started toilet-training and your child has just become dry during the day, this may cause them some toilet confusion at bedtime as they have used the toilet all day without 'wetting themselves' – which is how it now feels when they pee in the nappy. My advice is not to put on the nappy directly after their bath but to leave it off until after brushing their teeth and doing the last toilet run, directly before getting into bed, explaining, 'Just in case you pee while you're asleep, the nappy will hold it all in and you can take it off in the morning.'

If you then put your toddler to bed and he insists he needs another pee, you will have to judge how to manage this situation. Ask yourself: did he do a pee in the toilet before bed? Was it a substantial amount or was it just a tiny trickle? When did he last have a bigger pee? When did he last poop? If you're confident that he doesn't actually need to go at all, or are happy to stick with him using the nappy once it's 'sleepy-time', then just use your usual reassurances, remind him he's got his night-time nappy, ignore the demands and carry on with sleep-training.

You may decide to give him the benefit of the doubt and get him up just once to re-visit the toilet, but don't let him sit there for ages – if he really needs to go, he will do so quite quickly. Then put the nappy back in place and put him back to bed using the usual method. If he then calls out that he has had a pee in his nappy, my advice would be to ignore it and carry on with your usual reassurances until he goes to sleep. If indeed he has managed to squeeze out a 'protest poop', then obviously you will change him, but with minimal fuss and little interaction and putting him straight back to bed once you've changed him, continuing with the reassurance technique.

ALISON SAYS . . .

'Typically, children expel solid waste in the morning not in the middle of the night, so if your toddler is consistently pooping at random times throughout the night or at bedtime, I would suggest researching dietary issues and referring to Chapter 7 to see if there is a medical reason for this.'

Following this method, the evening toilet demands should quickly stop as your toddler responds to the firm boundaries you have established surrounding bed- and night-time.

Night-time toilet regressions

Toilet regressions – sudden bed-wetting or an unexpected night-time poop from a previously toilet-trained and dry-at-night toddler – are fairly common, and certainly challenging to deal with. The usual cause of a toilet regression at night is some kind of stress that your toddler has experienced. It might be due to something that happened earlier the same day, to an event that occurred a few days ago or even in response to something that hasn't yet happened! Perhaps your toddler had to go to the doctors the week before and had a procedure carried out – though you may think the event is over and done with, a sudden wet bed a week later could easily be a response to this upsetting experience. Equally, a toilet regression might occur in anticipation of a new sibling arriving or if there's been talk of your toddler moving to a new room at nursery or starting school.

It is always best to manage the 'accident' with as little fuss as possible and to settle him back down after a bed-change. Afterwards, don your 'baby detective' hat and try to work out what might be upsetting him.

If your toddler is of an age to understand, you could have a calm chat with him in the morning to see if he is aware of anything that is worrying him. However, avoid pushing him for answers as he might not even realize that he is feeling worried and that this is why he has wet the bed. Lots of re-assurance, positive attention and a protective sheet on the bed will all help, and hopefully it won't happen again.

If bed-wetting becomes repetitive, you will need to look further into the possible causes and check there's no underlying medical condition such as urinary tract infection. Speaking with your doctor or another specialist may also help if the problem is ongoing and you can't find a cause or resolution yourself.

☆ **ALISON'S GOLDEN RULES** ☆

1. Try not to worry about the effect that a new baby will have on your toddler. Millions of older siblings worldwide have to learn to accept the new family member.

2. Before the arrival of a new baby, give yourself plenty of time to work out who's going to sleep where and in what (cot in parents' room, first toddler bed etc.) and put into action any changes possible before the baby comes home.

3. If your little ones share a room, don't stress about them waking each other up – put the rules and boundaries in place and they will be fine.

4. Ask other family members for help at bath- and bedtime, when you have a new baby and a toddler or two to manage, all at the same time.

5. Persevere with your sleep-training for all the children, even it means you are going in and out of two or more bedrooms for an hour or so on the first night.

6. Plan ahead for how you are going to manage the UK's seasonal clock-change into your sleep-training.

7. Watch for signs that your toddler is ready to learn to be potty-trained and keep the transition simple and low-key.

8. Try not to be alarmed by any toilet 'accidents' and clear up with minimal fuss.

9. If you're travelling and your sleep routine regresses, don't panic – just enjoy your trip and know you can re-establish everything once you're home.

10. Remember that life often brings unexpected challenges and that disruptions to sleep can and do occur, but know that you always have the reassurance sleep-training technique to use as a tool to get things back on track.

CHAPTER 7

Reflux and Food Intolerances

In my first book, *The Sensational Baby Sleep Plan*, I dispelled the myths surrounding colic, explained the medical condition gastro-oesophageal reflux and detailed much information relating to cow's-milk-protein intolerance and allergy, including how to spot the symptoms of these digestive issues, how to find solutions and how to get a proper diagnosis. So you may ask why I am still talking about reflux and dietary intolerances in a book about toddlers' sleep, as it is generally taken that children grow out of these problems by twelve months of age . . . Wrong! From my years of experience working with babies, toddlers and young children, I can attest that many of them don't. Instead, as babies get older, they become somehow better able to 'self-manage' their discomfort and certainly don't show the same symptoms in response to their pain as they did during the first few months. This makes it easy to believe that they've simply outgrown the problem and that any issues they still have are due to developmental leaps, sleep regressions, general toddler behaviour or other expected life changes. So, again, many toddlers – just like babies – are not understood and any challenging behaviours they display are simply dismissed as being part of 'normal' toddlerhood!

The most frustrating problem that I've dealt with over the past twenty-five years working with non-sleeping toddlers is when they have an evident and obvious digestive issue, and related dietary intolerance or allergy, that has been misdiagnosed – or failed to be noticed at all. If a child has any degree of digestive discomfort or is experiencing pain from acid-reflux, they are obviously not going to be able to sleep soundly, but many are just labelled as poor sleepers, difficult children or tantruming toddlers.

To better understand what your child may be experiencing, it's worth knowing what's happening to the body with each of the conditions that may be causing the discomfort.

REFLUX EXPLAINED

The term reflux simply means 'backwards flow'. It is short for a condition called gastro-oesophageal reflux, or GOR, and is a physiological process in which the stomach contents are allowed to flow back up into the oesophagus. It occurs in everyone occasionally, young and old alike, although not everyone will feel any discomfort from it or even be aware that it is happening.

The oesophagus itself is a long, muscular tube that transports solid and liquid food from the mouth down to the stomach. It is connected to the stomach by a valve called the lower oesophageal sphincter, or LOS. This sphincter opens when you swallow to let food and drink pass through, and should then close to keep the stomach's contents inside. When the LOS doesn't function properly, however, it allows the stomach contents to flow back into the oesophagus to varying degrees. The contents may just flow into the lower end of the oesophagus (the distal), or may move further up towards the throat and sometimes enter the mouth and be ejected as vomit. Vomiting due to a physiological reflux of the stomach contents is much more common in younger babies, but certainly not unheard-of in toddlers or young children.

Basically, any degree of a 'backward flow' of the stomach contents can cause an acid heartburn, because the reflux material consists not only of the stomach contents but also a high level of hydrochloric acid. This acid is naturally produced in the stomach to aid the digestion of food, but while the stomach has a protective lining that acts as a barrier to the acid, the oesophagus does not. Over time, repeated exposure to the acid can cause severe pain, increasing damage to the oesophagus and sometimes more serious complications.

En route to the stomach, the oesophagus also connects to other openings, such as the trachea, or windpipe, and, at the back of the throat, to the sinuses, which lead to the nasal passages, and to the Eustachian tube, which leads to the middle ear along with a connection to the tear ducts. All of these passageways are linked and are lined with a mucosal membrane that, when in contact with gastric acid, will become irritated and inflamed. The passages therefore start to 'narrow' in places, and the only natural defence the body has is to secrete more mucus to try to flush away the acid and to soothe and repair the damage caused by the acid burn, which is why one symptom of acid-reflux is a snotty baby or toddler with a persistent cough.

The majority of babies are born with some degree of reflux simply from the immaturity of the lower oesophageal sphincter. Although many of them will not experience any pain or heartburn, and will indeed outgrow the condition within a few months without the need for medical intervention, sadly many others suffer severe discomfort and will need a medical diagnosis and an ongoing management plan for the condition and appropriate medical treatment. However, for babies, toddlers and children who do not 'grow out of it', the condition can then become a much more complex problem to resolve as there will be months, if not years, of acid damage, learned associations, pain-driven responses and psychological and emotional issues. After all, they have been self-managing a painful condition that they themselves aren't aware of – as it's just 'normal' to them because they have lived with it since birth and know no different!

SIGNS AND SYMPTOMS OF REFLUX AND INTOLERANCES IN OLDER BABIES AND TODDLERS

There are many indications that your child may be struggling with digestive issues, acid-reflux and dietary intolerances or food allergies, but the signs and symptoms can often be missed or misdiagnosed. The main problem is that every child will present with different symptoms and display different behaviours in response to the discomfort they feel from these conditions. Much depends on the severity of the condition. Symptoms can also differ depending on the child's temperament and also on environmental and social factors – all of which can make it harder to decipher what is actually going on.

Many parents are advised to wait for certain milestones when it is thought that their baby will just 'outgrow' the problem, but sadly this is rarely the case. For example, a GP may advise to start introducing solids earlier than normally recommended as it will help combat acid-reflux symptoms, but this is not always effective because the stomach then has more to digest, so food can actually exacerbate symptoms.

The following is a list of the most common physical symptoms and behavioural issues that toddlers may display or experience in response to acid-reflux, digestive discomfort, food intolerances and allergies.

- **Struggles to sleep** Lying down for periods of time can exacerbate reflux issues as acid seeps into the oesophagus. Your child may have failed to learn to sleep well as a baby due to their reflux pain and reluctance to lie down. It is possible she used to sleep OK but that the introduction of solids made the reflux worse, so she is now simply too uncomfortable to sleep.

- **Hates bedtime** Your toddler may have decided she doesn't like the long, lonely nights as she feels so uncomfortable and associates going to bed with night-time pain.

- **Wakes up screaming, crying or upset** Even if she does go to sleep, whenever she wakes she will cry as she's in pain from acid that's been building up while she's been lying down.

- **Never cries in the night, but just stays awake for hours** Some children give up crying in response to the discomfort but just lie awake for hours at night, fiddling with a comforter, chatting to themselves or even singing!

- **Won't nap in the day** She may seem to sleep OK at night, but has never been a good 'napper' and still refuses to sleep during the day.

- **Hot and sweaty at night** When we experience pain, our bodies produce extra adrenaline, which makes us hot and sweaty. (NB: When we are in pain, our sympathetic nerves trigger an adrenaline-powered 'fight or flight' response that simultaneously stimulates our sweat glands.)

- **'Mouth-breathes', often snores or has sleep apnoea** A child may have to breathe through her mouth when asleep due to acid damage in the throat, nasal passages and sinuses, and the consequent swelling and enlargement of the adenoids and tonsils. This may also cause her to snore or even briefly stop breathing while asleep (sleep apnoea). If ever you're worried about these issues, you could put an under-mattress breathing sensor in place.

- **Calls, cries out or talks in their sleep** Due to the child's constant feeling of discomfort, her brain remains more active and she may even shout out or cry in her sleep; sleep-talking is often a stress-related symptom. This level of brain activity also stops the body from going into a deep sleep so the child is never full rested.

- **Seems to be a very 'light' sleeper** Because her discomfort prevents her from going into a deep sleep, even the slightest noise wakes her up.

- **Is very restless when asleep and seems tired in the day** Even when she appears to be asleep, internal discomfort causes the toddler to thrash around, be constantly moving and end up in odd positions in the cot or bed. This means that the sleep she does have is not properly restful, so she's always tired.

- **Is a fussy eater** If a child learns that eating leads to discomfort or pain, they will shy away from it if possible. They will often only eat a few staple items of food, become phobic of trying anything new and be incredibly stubborn about what they will or won't eat. This learned association of food control can stay with them for life.

- **Overeats or constantly wants a snack** A toddler may look to eat small amounts throughout the day not because they are hungry, but because the food pushes down the acid and soothes their discomfort. This can lead to an ingrained association that food gives them comfort, which can cause problems in later life.

- **Refuses to give up milk in the night** Even though your toddler is over a year old, it may still seem that nothing will soothe your toddler back to sleep after a night-time waking except a breast- or bottle-feed. This is because your child has learned to use the milk to wash away the acid-reflux pain.

- **Is obsessed with the dummy** Sucking can help wash down the rising acid and therefore some toddlers are totally addicted to their dummy as it has become something they rely on to help with their pain.

- **Drinks excessive amounts of water** Many toddlers learn that water will help to wash food down their sore oesophagus, so they drink tons of water with each meal or want water throughout the night to help wash away acid pain.

- **Refuses to drink water** Some toddlers come to realize that drinking liquids makes their reflux worse, so they simply refuse to do it.

- **Can never seem to sit still and always runs everywhere** Similar to the agitation at night, and again in response to acid-reflux pain, some toddlers just cannot sit still. They are always 'on the go' and often run instead of walking, almost as if they are trying to escape their pain.

- **Will not sit still at mealtimes** Some children can become phobic about meals as they know eating makes them feel uncomfortable, so they are constantly getting up and down from the table to avoid eating. Often this leads to parents chasing the child all day with bits of food to try to get them to eat.

- **Will only eat with a distraction** Many parents become so desperate to get their food-resistant toddlers to eat that distraction, such as watching a screen, is the only way to get food into them. Once the child has 'zoned in' to the distraction, they are better able to absent-mindedly swallow food.

- **Has weight issues** Some children want to eat all the time to push down the pain from the acid, and therefore put on too much weight, whereas others struggle to eat in response to their pain and don't put on weight as one would expect.

- **Seems to have a very short attention span** Your child may often seem unable to concentrate on a particular task and have a very short attention span because she is always focusing on her internal discomfort. This means she is unable to sit and focus on a jigsaw, for example.

- **Has bowel issues** More often than not, if your child suffers with any degree of food intolerance or allergy they will either have loose, mushy stools, will poop too often or be constipated and unable to poop easily. Passing bowel movements in the night would also indicate that the digestive system might not be working as it should. A possible cause of this is too much fruit late in the day, but it could also be an intolerance or allergy.

- **Displays aggressive behaviour** At times, your toddler's pain may cause her to act aggressively when this isn't actually her temperament. Instead, she is simply displaying frustration at being in discomfort all the time.

- **Throws a tantrum at the slightest frustration** Your little one will often seem irrational and have total breakdowns at the slightest problem, simply because she cannot control her emotions as she is always feeling uncomfortable.

- **Almost self-harms by head-banging, scratching themselves or pulling their own hair** It is not unusual for toddlers to turn their aggressive feelings inward and harm themselves, rather than others, in response to their pain.

- **Has bad breath** Sometimes you will notice that your toddler has bad breath, especially in the morning. It might smell of vinegar or somewhat acidic, and if they suck their thumb or a comforter that may smell odd too.

- **Is congested and has a persistent cold or cough**
The body produces mucus in response to acid damage,
so your toddler may always seem congested or to have a
cold, a persistent cough or a constantly snotty nose.
A cow's-milk-protein intolerance will also cause the body
to create more mucus. Such children can often develop
chest infections due to the constant build-up of mucus.
The airways can become so sensitive that the child
wheezes and struggles to breathe; this is often diagnosed
as asthma, but the asthma medication doesn't seem to
help.

- **Has a hoarse or raspy voice** The vocal cords and voice
box can be damaged by the acid and cause a dry, hoarse
speaking tone.

- **Is delayed with their speech** If acid causes throat
discomfort when a child speaks, they are likely to
choose to stay silent and do not practise language skills.

- **Has dry skin, eczema or rashes** A toddler will often
have really dry skin, either all over the body, or in
patches. They may have 'bobbly' skin on their arms or
legs, or rashes that flare up. Such children are prescribed
creams to 'fix' the problem, but these only treat the
symptom, not the cause, which is often a cow's-milk-
protein intolerance or allergy.

- **Flushes red in the face and neck, especially when
eating** This happens because there is so much acid in
the oesophagus that as soon as they eat, the 'burn' from
the acid inside actually causes a red flush to the face
and neck.

- **Seems 'wired' and almost hyperactive** Typically, this
is because the toddler will not be sleeping well and is

herefore overtired, which manifests in some degree of hyperactivity. This may also be due to the excess adrenaline produced in response to being in pain.

- **Has recurring ear or throat infections** Nearly all ENT (ear, nose and throat) issues in babies, toddlers and young children are a result of acid damage from reflux. The majority of children who end up with glue ear and need to have grommets inserted will have suffered from acid-reflux.

- **Still vomits or spits up, even when on solid food** When young babies vomit or spit up, it's usually deemed normal, with many such children labelled as 'happy chuckers'. However, I don't believe it's normal in any way, and when they are still vomiting after introducing solids, the longer-term damage can be much more problematic.

- **Gags and chokes on food** Due to acid damage, they can often have a sensitive gag reflex and find swallowing difficult. This can cause them to gag on food and have frequent choking episodes.

- **'Food-crams'** Your toddler may often put much too much food into her mouth in one go so she doesn't have to keep swallowing smaller mouthfuls, but she will often then just let the food fall out of her mouth as she can't swallow the amount she has put in.

- **Has severe reactions to teething** Every bout of teething seems to be hugely problematic as their body is already so focused on trying to cope with its digestive issues that there's no energy left to deal with other causes of pain. Teething also creates excess acid in the gut, which hugely exacerbates the acid-reflux problem already there.

- **Seems to want to climb everything** These children can often be seen scaling sofas, chairs, tables, furniture – and even you! It's almost as if they want to climb away from their pain.

- **Displays repetitive or obsessive behaviours** Being able to distract themselves, for example, opening and closing a cupboard door that makes a loud bang as they slam it shut, can help them forget about their internal discomfort.

- **Is often very loud and vocal** You toddler may often shout or squeal, and no matter how much you try and get them to be quieter, they simply can't do it as they've learned to make lots of noise as a distraction from their pain.

- **Walks on tiptoes** Many of the children who suffer with acid-reflux will walk on their tiptoes and seem to always want to stretch upwards, away from their discomfort. They also seem to not like pressure on their feet, and don't like wearing socks or shoes.

- **Dislikes getting their hands dirty** Your toddler may often hold their arms out to the sides, waving their hands in the air when they are walking, to avoid getting anything on them.

- **Is hugely stubborn, determined and difficult to manage** Living with internal discomfort can cause these children to develop stubborn personality traits because they learn very quickly what makes them feel slightly more comfortable and will become extremely resistant to anything that doesn't.

- **Is very picky about what clothes they will wear** You may have huge battles over what clothes they will wear and what they won't. It's all about control over what they feel comfortable with, and often they don't actually like the feeling of wearing clothes at all, as their internal discomfort makes their nerve endings seem highly sensitive.

- **Struggles to interact with other children** The child is so focused on coping with their condition that they have little patience for social interactions with other children – they can often seem stand-offish and even be quite aggressive to other playmates.

- **Doesn't listen or seems to ignore you** She may often seem to be in her own little world and appear not to hear or listen to you, and won't answer, because she is just so internally focused on her discomfort.

- **Is travel-sick** Many children who have travel sickness actually have acid-reflux and their gut just can't cope with the addition of the unnatural motion of a car.

The list of symptoms is vast and it's almost impossible that any child would display all of the ones I've given here, and in many cases the symptoms will differ from child to child depending on various other factors as previously mentioned.

You may have noticed that many of the symptoms listed above are similar to those linked to hyperactivity, ADHD and autistic behaviours. I have worked with many children who have been diagnosed either with some kind of learning disability, as being 'somewhere on the spectrum', as 'late-learners' or having a 'sensory processing disorder' or 'compulsive behavioural disorder'. While I don't discount these conditions, in the majority of cases I've come across, the children don't have any of these disorders or conditions; instead, their behaviours are driven by, and are in response to, being in pain from acid-reflux or a food intolerance, both of which cause them untold internal discomfort. In addition, many children with reflux never sleep easily, comfortably or properly and therefore experience a high degree of sleep deprivation. However, once these issues have been properly understood and managed, the children start to sleep better and no longer display their difficult, odd and frustrating behaviours, instead transforming into much calmer and happier little people!

A PARENT'S STORY

'We asked Alison to come and help with our three-month-old baby, but while with us she also helped with our older daughter, Sophia, who was nearly four years old. As a young toddler, Sophia hadn't crawled, stood up or walked. She didn't vocalize or say words; she only cried. She didn't climb a stair, jump or pull toys along. Her eating habits were odd: she craved food and massively overate, though as she got older she would only eat with distraction from a screen; she never moved on to "normal" food and would only eat food mashed up together – with no lumps! Not a single health professional looked at these and the other odd behaviours our daughter had displayed since infancy (so many of which we now know are typical of reflux), and mostly we had been dismissed, with everything classed as being "normal". We simply found a way to cope and "manage" our little girl. We got her into a vague routine and implemented a bath- and bedtime. This helped but it was always fraught, challenging and not the calm peaceful end-of-day one hopes for.

She was also a light sleeper, was hot and sweaty throughout the night, and would thrash and kick out in her cot. She was always extremely tired throughout the day as the quality of her sleep was so poor, but we could never understand why this was the case.

Sophia began taking steps soon after her second birthday, and, at nearly four, she had a complete range of movement. But one of the biggest problems as Sophia got older was managing her challenging behaviour. She developed an almost aggressive response to simple requests, would lash out, hit, throw things and have complete meltdowns at the slightest thing. We found ways to get through these tantrums – and there could be many in one day – but it's been completely and utterly exhausting for us all.

The onerous label of "development delay" was bestowed upon her, but sadly without any real testing or proper assessment to back it up, and seemingly without any real understanding of her condition.

When we first sat with Alison and told her the whole sorry story, we were amazed at the questions Alison asked us as they related to all the things that we had questioned over the past few years. Alison spent time observing Sophia and became absolutely certain that our daughter had experienced severe reflux as a baby and had suffered with a cow's-milk-protein allergy and that she had never grown out of it!

The next day we all went to see a paediatric gastroenterologist who, after much discussion, 100 per cent concurred with Alison. The consultant prescribed Sophia omeprazole, which reduces acid in the stomach, and advised putting her on a dairy- and soya-free diet, as well as avoiding wheat and gluten.

After just over two months on omeprazole and her allergen-free diet, Sophia is so much better in every respect. Her sleep is now undisturbed. Her behaviour changed dramatically, too, and although she still tends to get cross quite quickly, it rarely escalates into a full-blown tantrum.

We are so thankful for the day Alison walked into – and changed – our lives.'

E. D.-L.

FOOD INTOLERANCES AND ALLERGIES

Acid-reflux is a simple backward flow of the stomach contents, but it can often be caused or exacerbated by food intolerances or allergies. A food 'allergy' is an abnormal response by the body's immune system to a certain food. This is different from a food 'intolerance', which does not affect the immune system, although some of the same symptoms may be present. If a food allergy or intolerance is driving the acid-reflux, knowing this will help with managing the reflux and bringing it under control.

Lactose intolerance: the basics

Lactose intolerance is the inability of the stomach to digest significant amounts of lactose, which is a complex sugar found in milk. People sometimes confuse lactose intolerance with cow's-milk-protein intolerance because the two conditions, while quite separate, can induce similar symptoms. An allergy can cause similar symptoms but is due to an immune-system response, rather than a primarily digestive one, and can affect any number of organs in the body. The symptoms can also be more extreme, such as anaphylactic shock, which can be life-threatening.

Lactose intolerance is due to a shortage of the enzyme lactase, which is needed to break down the lactose in the milk. If the digestive system is deficient in lactase, the symptoms can include:

- excess bloating

- trapped wind

- stomach cramps

- explosive, green, loose and watery stools

A lactose intolerance can also occur after a gastro-intestinal infection or tummy bug, and can last for up to six weeks. Sometimes vaccines or ingesting certain medicines can also cause a temporary lactose intolerance.

Few children actually have a genuine problem with lactose, though in some cases it can indicate that there might be a more serious underlying cause, such as Crohn's disease, coeliac disease or inflammatory bowel disease.

Cow's-milk-protein intolerance and allergy: the basics

Cow's-milk-protein allergy (CMPA) is the most common food allergy in babies and children. Although it is estimated to affect more than 2 per cent of children under the age of three, I believe there are many more children who are never actually diagnosed. It is also suggested that most children with the allergy will typically outgrow it by the age of five, but I have found this is not always the case and have worked with many older children who have had longer-term problems due to a cow's-milk allergy they have never grown out of.

CMPA occurs when the body's immune system reacts abnormally to a protein in the milk of cows and some other animals. Normally, the immune system protects our bodies from harmful pathogens like bacteria and viruses. In CMPA, the immune system mistakes a protein in cow's milk as a harmful substance and attacks it. This immune reaction can damage the baby's or child's stomach and intestines. Proteins found in some beans, most noticeably the soya bean, have a similar structure to that of cow's-milk protein and therefore many children with a cow's-milk-protein allergy may also be sensitive to soya-bean protein. Allergy testing can often pinpoint an individual's sensitivity to other proteins and food groups.

The allergic reaction to milk can begin within minutes of ingesting it or it can be delayed for several hours; sometimes it can be days or even weeks before a reaction is noticeable, especially if there is only an intolerance to the milk protein, and not a full-blown allergy. Symptoms may include:

- stomach pain

- nausea

- acid-reflux

- diarrhoea

- constipation

- erratic bowel movements

- skin rashes

- eczema

- swelling of the lips or throat

- upper respiratory congestion

- trouble breathing

If you suspect your child has any form of cow's-milk issue, it is best to completely remove all dairy and soy products from his diet for a short time and watch for any changes, reactions or improvements in symptoms. If there is a significant positive change then you might assume that your child does have some sort of issue with most cow's-milk products and it would be wise to keep the diet dairy-free for another few weeks before perhaps reintroducing some dairy very gradually, to see if there's any further reaction. Often, just by giving the system a break, your child may well be able to go back to having dairy in his diet; this may need to remain at a restricted level or he may be able to tolerate a full dairy-inclusive diet once more.

However, if removing milk doesn't seem to have improved his symptoms, before reintroducing the cow's milk I would advise keeping his diet dairy-free for a while longer and removing gluten as well. It is sometimes necessary to remove all dairy, soya, and gluten before there is an improvement in symptoms, and after this break from all major allergens it will become clearer which, if any – or even all – are causing the problems.

Gluten intolerance and allergy: the basics

Intolerance to gluten – a protein found in wheat, barley and rye – is becoming increasingly prevalent and affects babies, children, teens and adults alike. The most severe form of gluten intolerance is coeliac disease, an auto-immune condition that affects about 1 per cent of the population and can lead to permanent damage to the digestive system. There is a higher percentage of people with a non-coeliac gluten sensitivity (NCGS) – a recent study showed that an estimated 13 per cent of the population in the UK suffer with this condition.

Both forms of gluten intolerance can cause widespread symptoms, many of which have nothing to do with digestion, but these are the main signs and symptoms of gluten intolerance:

- bloating and excess bottom-wind, which can be very smelly

- diarrhoea or very wet, mushy and sometimes smelly stools

- constipation and often smelly stools

- abdominal pain, tummy aches and stomach cramps

- headaches and migraines

- fatigue and lack of energy

- skin problems such as psoriasis and alopecia

- mood swings, depression and anxiety

- unexpected weight loss

- iron-deficiency (anaemia)

- auto-immune disorders

- joint and muscle pain, or numbness and pins and needles in arms and legs

- 'brain fog' and inability to focus

In my opinion, gluten intolerance is much more prevalent than is generally understood, and often the medical problems it causes are diagnosed and treated only as individual conditions, without the root cause, of gluten allergy or intolerance, ever being realized.

CAUSES OF FOOD ALLERGIES AND INTOLERANCES

According to NAFA (Natasha Allergy Research Foundation), in the UK 6–8 per cent of children up to the age of three years have food allergies. The prevalence of reported food allergies is definitely on the increase, and although most children 'outgrow' their allergies at some point, allergies to peanuts, tree nuts, fish and shellfish can be life-long.

To become allergic to a food, a child must have been exposed to the food at least once before her first reaction to it, even through breast milk after the mother has eaten the food. It is the second time the child eats the food that the allergic symptoms appear. This time, when antibodies react with the food, histamine is released, which can cause the child to experience hives, asthma, itching in the mouth, trouble breathing, stomach pains, vomiting and/or diarrhoea. The symptoms can be merely uncomfortable or they can be life-threatening.

(NB: Histamine is produced when the body's defence and protection mechanism – the immune system – believes that the body has been exposed to a harmful substance, at which point it emits signals that cause the release of this chemical into the bloodstream. An unfortunate side effect is that histamine irritates areas like the eyes, nose, throat, lungs or gastrointestinal tract, causing the allergy symptoms. Antihistamine medication is used to treat allergy symptoms as it reduces the amount of histamine produced by the body.)

Approximately 90 per cent of all food allergies are caused by the following eight foods:

- milk

- eggs

- wheat

- soy

- tree nuts

- peanuts

- fish

- shellfish

Eggs, milk, peanuts, wheat, soy and tree nuts are the most common causes of food allergies in children, with the most severe reactions caused by peanuts, tree nuts, fish and shellfish.

The tendency to develop allergies is often hereditary, which means it can be passed down through the genes, from parents to their children. However, just because you, your partner or one of your children might have allergies, it doesn't mean that all of your children will definitely get them (although the likelihood is higher), and some children have allergies even if no other family member is allergic. Unfortunately, those who are allergic to one thing are likely to be allergic to others. There are, of course, non-food allergies too, such as those to pollen, dust mites, pets and mould, plus insect bites, latex, certain chemicals, sulphites and medicines; even penicillin contains allergens that can cause a reaction.

DIAGNOSING FOOD INTOLERANCES AND ALLERGIES

It is always advisable to seek medical help for suspected allergies or intolerances, and in the majority of cases a preliminary diagnosis can be made based on the symptoms your child is displaying. If there is any suspicion that he has some underlying digestive discomfort, you may need to remove a particular type of food, or even all of them in turn, for a trial period to see if things improve or not.

If you have unsuccessfully tried to reintroduce certain food groups, further medical help will be needed and your child may need some proper allergy tests carried out. There are a number of tests available although they are not routinely offered.

- **Hydrogen breath test** Undigested lactose produces high levels of hydrogen gas in the breath. Doctors can diagnose lactose intolerance by measuring the hydrogen level after you drink a lactose-loaded beverage.

- **Stool acidity test** Undigested lactose increases the amount of acid in the stool. Doctors may test a sample to diagnose lactose intolerance in young children.

- **Food-allergy testing** If your doctor suspects a milk allergy, you may be sent to an allergist for skin-prick testing or have a blood sample taken for laboratory allergy testing.

Bear in mind that a mild intolerance to a particular allergen might not always show up in testing, even though it obviously causes a reaction in your child.

Sometimes there is no available test, such as with a histamine intolerance, and the only way to find a resolution is through removing certain foods and charting the reactions or changes.

Your doctor may refer you to an allergy specialist and a dietician, who can then advise you on how best to avoid a particular food allergen while still maintaining good nutrition for your child. You could also seek help from a nutritionist, who can advise on what foods to try or to eliminate, and how to promote a healthy gut microbiome – the bacteria and other organisms that maintain gut health – such as by using probiotics to help repair a gut that has been damaged by a food allergy.

ANTIBIOTICS AND COW'S-MILK-PROTEIN INTOLERANCE

Antibiotics are essential to cure infections but they have a hugely negative effect on gut flora that can spark off an allergic reaction to foods. A research paper published by the National Library for Medicine concludes that both mothers' and their offspring's use of antibiotics were associated with an increased risk of cow's-milk allergy. When babies and children are exposed to antibiotics – while still in the womb, during birth, through breast milk or given directly – the developing gut microbiome is damaged and this can cause an intolerance or allergy. I'm not suggesting that antibiotics shouldn't be used when necessary, but extra care and advice from the prescribing doctor should be given on how to lessen the impact for a little one's gut, by taking prebiotics or probiotics, for example.

MANAGING DIETARY CHANGES FOR YOUR CHILD

It can be quite a daunting prospect to change your toddler's diet, if that is what's required to overcome digestive problems. That said, it is much easier today than it was ten or fifteen years ago, when you could only get gluten-free products on prescription. Today, all the supermarkets have a large 'free-from' range and a multitude of plant- and nut-based milks readily available, for example, and there is plenty of information from trusted sources online on how to keep a healthy and balanced diet for toddlers despite dietary changes.

There is much more awareness surrounding food allergies and intolerances, and a plethora of information available online about adopting a dairy-free, gluten-free or vegan diet. For instance, there are hundreds of social media groups you can join that will give you information on the best alternative brands and allergen-free recipes, along with advice, help and support with whatever changes you are needing to make. Meanwhile, nearly all food outlets, restaurants, cafes, schools and nurseries now cater for food allergies, so thankfully it's not quite the minefield it used to be. However, you will still need to read the labels on everything you buy, as there can be 'hidden' ingredients in some prepared foods and it's sometimes easy to be confused by the wording.

For example, when needing to adopt a dairy-free diet, you'll need to know that all of the following terms indicate that milk, or derivatives of milk, are present in the food:

- cow's milk (fresh, UHT, malted, evaporated and condensed)

- dried milk, skimmed milk powder

- milk solids, non-fat milk solids, milk protein

- butter, butter oil, buttermilk, ghee

- cream, sour cream

- cheese, cream cheese, curd cheese, quark

- yoghurt, fromage frais, crème fraîche

- casein, casein concentrate, hydrolysed casein, casein hydrolysate, sodium caseinate, ammonium caseinate or magnesium caseinate

- lactose, lactoglobulin, lactulose, lactalbumin, lactalbumin phosphate, lactoacidophilus

- whey, hydrolysed whey, whey powder, whey syrup sweetener, whey protein hydrolysate, sweet whey, delactosed whey

'THEY JUST GROW OUT OF IT, DON'T THEY?'

The idea that children grow out of food intolerances is an interesting one. While many intolerances and allergies will improve over time, as a baby's gut matures, I know from experience that in many cases these problems can actually get worse. I've had many parents contact me thinking that their toddler's sleep problems had been caused by a predictable sleep regression or a developmental leap, but instead of it being the short-term issue it was supposed be, things just escalated and have continued to get worse. In many cases this is due to a food intolerance or allergy that has caused increasing digestive distress and discomfort and that prevents the child from sleeping and just gets worse over time.

Meanwhile, for some babies who have an intolerance or sensitivity to cow's-milk protein, this may not be apparent until the parents wean them from breastfeeding or the baby's usual formula to cow's milk at twelve months, following NHS advice. However, it is highly unlikely that such an allergy would have remained completely unnoticed before this, given that the baby would already have started solids.

A PARENT'S STORY

'I followed Alison's plan as soon as my daughter was born, and from thirteen weeks she slept through the night. However, she had often seemed a bit restless at night and had an irritating cough that nothing seemed to cure. At around fourteen months she started to wake during the night and by fifteen months she was crying and screaming at bedtime. I literally had no clue what was wrong, so I called Alison. After asking me a multitude of questions, Alison deduced that my daughter was not coping with the cow's milk that I had introduced soon after she turned one. In hindsight, and with Alison's explanation, I realized that the restlessness at night had increased at eight months, when I had stopped breastfeeding and switched to formula; after the change to cow's milk at twelve months her sleep had just deteriorated even further. Because the reaction wasn't immediate, I hadn't put two and two together! Alison explained that my daughter had a cow's-milk-protein intolerance and it was causing her much digestive discomfort, which would continue to get worse. I immediately removed all dairy, and within four nights my daughter was back to sleeping through the night! Now two-and-a-half years old, my daughter now has some dairy in her diet (in moderation) and she's totally fine.'

S. L.

Gluten intolerance can also develop over time, as your toddler starts to eat a wider variety of foods and because so many of these contain high levels of gluten. Gluten is a key culprit of night-time waking in young children, but is rarely identified as such. As you start to wean your baby on to lovely vegetables, and then to introduce proteins and carbohydrates, your toddler's diet becomes increasingly gluten-rich. Having displayed no immediate reaction when you introduced bread or pasta products, for example, when your toddler suddenly stops sleeping at night no one would think to link it to a gluten sensitivity. But by the time your toddler is fourteen months old, he might be eating Weetabix and toast for breakfast, sandwiches or wraps for lunch and a pasta dish for supper, all of which are heavily laden with gluten, which can cause pain in the sensitive gut and therefore interfere with his sleep.

Another big problem is that a vast number of foods contain gluten without most buyers realizing it, unless they read the labels in minute detail – such as sausages, chips, processed white-potato products, gravies, ketchup, soy sauce and salad dressings, processed cold meats, sweets and most dry snacks. It is therefore very easy for a diet to contain high levels of gluten and it is causing huge problems for many of today's toddlers and young children.

MEDICATIONS

Acid-reflux may well need treatment from a paediatric gastro-enterologist or doctor, who might prescribe an acid suppressant such as omeprazole.

Omeprazole is from a group of medicines called proton pump inhibitors (PPIs) and they work by shutting down the acid pumps in the stomach, which then reduces the gastric acid secretion. This then helps stop the backward flow of the stomach contents and therefore reduces the burning pain caused by acid in the oesophagus.

FINDING RESOLUTION

In many older babies and toddlers, the primary condition that is causing the digestive issue is often a food intolerance or allergy of some kind. It is this that creates the acid-reflux problem, which is actually the secondary condition and only a symptom of the food allergy. For this reason, the use of omeprazole need only be a short-term solution, as the removal of the food group causing the allergy or intolerance will allow the gut to heal and repair itself over time. Nonetheless, the use of omeprazole to reduce gastric acid, alongside the new diet, in many cases also allows the damage to the oesophagus and all the mucosal 'pipes' to heal more quickly. This will mean the child experiences much more relief and comfort in a shorter space of time, rather than just waiting for everything to heal in the longer term. This will have the knock-on effect of you being able to encourage better sleep associations for your toddler and implement the reassurance sleep-training accordingly.

This whole scenario of gut health and how it affects sleep can be complex to understand, but increasing research suggests that the brain and the gut are strongly connected, that one has an effect on the other and that poor sleep can negatively affect your gut microbiome, which in turn can lead to additional health issues, including an increased risk of gastro-oesophageal reflux.

The gut microbiome is the term for all the microorganisms found in your gastrointestinal tract and stomach, such as bacteria, viruses, protozoa and fungi. Understanding the correlation between the gut and sleep is all very well, but you can't expect a child who is uncomfortable due to digestive issues to sleep properly! However, there is much that can be done if you realize your toddler has been uncomfortable for some time due to battling a food intolerance and has had acid-reflux as a result. Once you have sought medical help and feel that your child is more comfortable, you can finally implement the sleep-training. That said, in many cases very little sleep-training is actually needed as the child is so relieved not to be in discomfort that they just sleep!

BEDTIME AND SLEEP FOR A TODDLER WITH REFLUX

If your child has been experiencing digestive problems and acid-reflux for some time and is displaying some of the signs and symptoms previously described, it is highly likely she will have developed strongly negative associations with sleep. Her reactions to being in discomfort, and consequently her inability to sleep comfortably, will be so deeply ingrained that they may well be hard to change, but with careful management and understanding it can be done.

ALISON SAYS . . .

'I took a call from some parents with an eighteen-month-old who still repeatedly woke during the night. He had never slept well as a young baby and had "colic" issues in the first few months, so his mum, who was breastfeeding, ended up co-sleeping as the baby simply would not be put down and just wanted to be attached to her – literally! She explained that at six months she had tried to implement some sleep-training but he had just screamed and screamed so she gave up. At ten months, she managed to wean him off the breast and on to cow's milk, but he then got eczema so she switched to oat milk. He continued to wake and cry for milk all through the night, and though she managed to remove the endless bottles by sixteen months, he still didn't sleep!

Since his mum had never been able to get him to go into a cot, he slept in a double bed in his own room, but once he woke he wouldn't go back to sleep unless his mum slept with him, so most nights his mum ended up just sleeping in with him until the morning. The situation was hugely stressful and was putting an immense strain on family relationships.

The toddler also had erratic but frequent mushy poops and bloated tummy, and he often passed smelly wind. He also thrashed around all over the bed when sleeping.

My explanation, of a likely gluten intolerance and, consequently, an acid-reflux issue, was somewhat surprising to the parents, but after much discussion they began to understand my thinking. After getting omeprazole prescribed and removing gluten from the toddler's diet, things were already much improved, but he still wanted to sleep with Mum. This was totally understandable, as he had always used the comfort of his mum to help him manage his discomfort so his association and desire to be with her was deeply ingrained. After much careful consideration, we organized a pillow with a photo of Mummy on it and a sleep-clock, then devised some bedtime rules ready for sleep-training. I advised changing the bed from a double to a single so there "wouldn't be room" for Mummy to lie down with him, and within four nights he was going to sleep alone and self-settling if he woke. Another huge success story!'

Whatever extreme reactions your toddler displays, especially surrounding sleep, please rest assured that they can be altered and that calmer, more peaceful nights can be achieved. However, you may need to adapt certain aspects of the sleep-training to accommodate your individual toddler and be ever-mindful of his diet, ensuring that it remains appropriately free from any foods causing an allergy or intolerance.

MEALTIMES FOR A TODDLER WITH REFLUX

Many toddlers who have suffered with, or are currently still experiencing, acid-reflux symptoms can display quite 'odd' behaviours when weaning on to solids. For example, your toddler may have:

- point-blank refused to open their mouth for solids
- eaten the food but looked uncomfortable afterwards
- decided food is better than milk, then started refusing milk feeds
- only eaten tiny amounts – or almost too much
- started eating solid food with enthusiasm, but after a few weeks decided they don't like it
- become resistant to spoon-feeding and only want the food they can eat themselves or that you can feed them with your fingers
- never progressed past the purée stage and refused to eat 'proper' food
- never accepted the lumpy-food stage in conventional weaning methods

- learned that the only way to eat food is to wash it down with copious amounts of water

- never wanted to sit in their designated high-chair as they don't like feeling restrained

- developed some odd and extreme body movements, perhaps contorting their arms and shoulders into weird positions and turning their head almost like an owl

The variety of responses is vast and is driven by individual personality traits, environmental factors and how well – or not – their reflux has been managed, and therefore how digestively comfortable they feel. These initial responses to food will often also lay the pathway for children's attitudes to solids for years to come and that is why many are labelled as 'fussy eaters' or 'grazers'. Some will continue to resist food whereas others crave food and want to eat all the time. What makes one child decide not to eat in response to acid-reflux and another want to eat all the time still remains a mystery to me!

ALISON SAYS . . .

'As a baby, my slightly older sister was a really "difficult" feeder. Our mum told us she never liked milk and would vomit after every feed. Her dislike of milk continued and carried over into her associations with food; Mum always described her as a "fussy eater". She never wanted to eat and I remember myself the battles they had at the dinner table, with her then being served for breakfast what she hadn't eaten for dinner the evening before!

Then along I came, and apparently I cried endlessly – except when I was being fed. I craved milk, and would have fed all the time if Mum had let me. Starting on solid food didn't change things much: I would eat as much as possible, soon being labelled and teased as being "greedy". I piled on weight and was obese as a child, whereas my sister remained pretty thin by comparison.

Our individual associations with milk and food in those early months have stayed with us for life. My sister has a slim figure and has never really struggled with any weight-gain, even after having two children. (Interestingly, however, she still easily vomits – one glass of wine too many, or some food that slightly doesn't agree, and she will continue to vomit for a day or two at a time, whereas I hardly ever vomit and never did as a baby.) Meanwhile, I have always eaten too much and struggled with being overweight. I also still battle to manage acid-reflux, and when I am anxious I reach for food as a comfort; I never lose weight, as many people do, in response to stress. There are many other things that I have experienced that I know are a result of suffering long-term acid-reflux, and it has certainly shaped my life. I sometimes wonder how different things might have been if my acid-reflux as an infant had been properly managed in those early days.'

Introducing solids and maintaining healthy associations with mealtimes for children who suffer from acid-reflux and dietary-related allergies or intolerances can be a painstaking process that will need careful management and great patience. In my opinion, there needs to be much more research into acid-reflux and the responses it induces in babies and toddlers, especially in relation to food, to provide parents with more information and support when trying to manage the condition in their little ones.

Practical tips for mealtimes

If you have a food-resistant toddler, mealtimes can be tricky to manage, and there is no single rule that works for all. As parents, but especially as mothers, our deepest, strongest and most naturally nurturing instinct is to feed our young. When our offspring don't want to feed, don't seem to like feeding and even scream or protest when we try to feed them, it produces such a huge mix of distressing maternal emotions – you may feel panic, frustration, despair and even anger. This means that feeds or mealtimes become stressful and challenging events that both mother and child almost fear, rather than the enjoyable, calm and social situations one would hope them to be.

The best way to manage this situation is probably the hardest to actually implement – and that is to relax! Of course, when your baby won't feed or your toddler won't eat the meal you've just cooked, the last thing in the world you feel is relaxed, and trying to manage and 'hide' all these raw emotions is incredibly difficult.

ALISON SAYS . . .

'Many years ago, I created a mental image to reflect the satisfaction we feel when our babies feed well. Imagine a baby's bottle full of milk and alongside a "maternal satisfaction-ometer". As the amount of milk in the bottle reduces, the "satisfaction-ometer" level rises, bringing about a huge feel-good factor, and almost a sense of relief, when we know our little one has had a good feed!'

Here are some top tips to help lower your stress levels and more easily manage the mealtimes:

- Turn on the radio or some music so you have a distraction to listen to or sing along with.

- Change the mealtime environment occasionally, perhaps by hosting a 'picnic' outside or sitting around a small table in another room.

- Invite friends round to coincide with a mealtime, to make things more enjoyable for you and provide a distraction for your child. Obviously they need to be the kind of friends who understand your situation and who you feel comfortable with even when things are stressful.

- Have other, happily-eating children come for mealtimes so your child can learn from their positive mealtime behaviour.

- Provide some physical distractions for the mealtime, such as toy food or wipe-clean books.

- Play audio-stories for your toddler to listen to while eating.

- Try to eat at the same time as your child and share food, rather than focus only on what he is eating.

- Resist the temptation to constantly encourage him to eat; it's actually better to say hardly anything about the food itself and instead just chit-chat about anything else you can think of.

- Try not to let your child know how anxious you feel and avoid watching his every mouthful. Give an impression of complete disinterest in how much he eats or doesn't eat.

- Avoid offering 'reward' food, such as pudding, if the main course is finished, or stating that one thing has to be eaten in order to 'earn' another.

- Set a time limit for the meal, and when the time is up clear away, no matter what's been eaten and what's left on your toddler's plate. You could get a timer to use for this and devise some 'mealtime rules' similar to the bedtime ones.

- Above all, make absolutely sure your toddler is digestively comfortable and that any reflux issues or food intolerances are being properly managed.

Managing a baby or toddler with reflux can be one of the most challenging tasks you ever have to undertake, and I sincerely hope that all the information in this chapter is of some help. Remember, you know your child better than anyone, and if you instinctively feel something is not quite right then seek help, ask questions and don't let anyone fob you off. Persevere until you find someone who will listen, who takes you seriously and who can provide the help and support you need.

☆ ALISON'S GOLDEN RULES ☆

1. If you instinctively feel that there is something wrong or not quite right with your toddler or child, trust your instincts and persevere with trying to find someone who will listen and be able to help.

2. If you suspect your child has a food intolerance, it can be useful to keep a food diary for a week or two to record his reactions.

3. Remember, when making dietary changes it can take time to see the full effects, so be patient.

4. Never 'force' your toddler to eat all his food as it will just make him more resistant to eating.

5. Remember that sleep-health is hugely important in managing acid-reflux and helping to repair and boost gut health.

6. Always ask for a second opinion and to be referred to another doctor or paediatrician if you're not happy with the advice or diagnosis from your current medical professional.

7. If your child has been exposed to antibiotics at any point, you can help to boost his gut health by giving pre- and probiotics.

8. If your child's sleep habits suddenly change, don't just accept that it's a developmental 'leap' or a 'regression,' but look more closely at what could be causing it, especially if you've recently introduced new foods or changed milks.

9. If your child is a very 'active' sleeper and thrashes around in the night, then it's highly likely he has some degree of digestive distress and possible food intolerance.

10. Managing a food-resistant toddler can be incredibly challenging, but remember that with the right understanding, diagnosis and help, things can and will improve!

If you are struggling with your toddler's sleep at present, please remember that life will not stay this way for ever. You have the tools you need for them to sleep solidly and to establish a routine that will serve you and your little one well for years to come. It can be nerve-wracking to take those initial steps, and particularly daunting when negative habits feel ingrained, but there is no reason that the advice in this book won't work for you, as it has for countless others.

If you think, having read this book, that your child may be struggling with reflux issues, rest assured that this can almost always be brought under control, and that it is easily possible to manage food intolerances. It is also easier than you might think to instil good sleep habits in your home. You have everything you need right here.

So now it's time to take that leap of faith and establish better sleep for your toddler – and for you!

Sources

Marsh, Sarah, 'Children's lack of sleep is "hidden health crisis", experts say', *Guardian*, 30 Sep 2018.

Stanford, Christie, 'To crib or not to crib', MariaMontessori.com, 10 July 2010.

Hicks, Tony, 'More teens need prescription glasses. Is excessive screen time to blame?', Healthline, 19 Aug 2019.

Griffin, R. Morgan, 'This is your kid's brain without sleep', WebMD.com, 1 May 2013.

'Sleep deprivation', Wikipedia.

HealthDay Reporter, 'Sleep deprivation and new parents', HealthDay, 31 Dec 2019.

Pelly, Julia, 'The 2-year-old sleep regression: what you should know', Healthline, 17 Apr 2020.

Sadeh, Avi, Gruber, Reut and Raviv, Amiram, 'The effects of sleep restriction and extension on school-age children: what a difference an hour makes', *Child Development*, 74(2), 2003, pp. 444–55.

Plowman, Val, 'Overstimulation for toddlers', Babywisemom.com, 3 Jan 2019.

'Delivering Effective Services for Children and Young People with ADHD', Greater Manchester Combined Authority, July 2015 (revised 2018).

Pacheco, Danielle, 'Children and Sleep', Sleep Foundation, 24 Sep 2020.

'Your child's sleep affects their brain', Children's Health.

'Overstimulation: babies and children', raisingchildren.net.au, 20 Oct 2020.

'Epigenetics and child development: how children's experiences affect their genes', Center on the Developing Child, Harvard University.

'Child Development: Toddlers (2–3 years of age)', Centers for Disease Control and Prevention, 22 Feb 2021.

Cassoff, Jamie, Gruber, Reut and Wiebe, Sabrina T., 'Sleep patterns and the risk for ADHD: a review', *Nature and Science of Sleep*, 4, 2012, pp. 73–80.

'Developmental and Emotional Milestones Leaflet', Our Place.

Fitzgerald, Louisa, 'Toddler growth and development', Verywell Family, 29 Jan 2020.

McCready, Amy, '10 tips for better behavior', Positive Parenting Solutions.

Deflin, Kendall, '10 positive benefits of listening to music, according to science', Live For Live Music, 17 Feb 2016.

Murkoff, Heidi, 'Growth and development month by month', What to Expect, 16 Jan 2019.

Coghill, David, Currie, Craig J., Holden, Sarah E., Jenkins-Johns, Sara, Morgan, Christopher L. I. and Poole, Chris D., 'The prevalence and incidence, resource use and financial costs of treating people with attention deficit/hyperactivity disorder (ADHD) in the United Kingdom (1998 to 2010)', *Child and Adolescent Psychiatry and Mental Health*, 7(34), 2013.

'Toddler sleep concerns: over-stimulation', Babycentre.

Munson, Joan, 'Attention-seeking behavior in young children: do's and don'ts for parents', Empowering Parents.

Gindin, Rona, 'What toddlers understand when adults talk', Parents.com, 18 Nov 2020.

Hood, Lauren, 'Establishing "pecking order" with your dog', *Unleash Magazine*.

'Sing and Sign . . . What is it?', singandsign.co.uk

'Five ways to teach your toddler manners', Babycentre.

Bickerstaff Glover, Robin, '11 helpful tips for teaching kids manners', *The Spruce*, 25 Mar 2020.

Bly, Jennifer, 'Setting boundaries for toddlers', Focus on the Family, 13 Oct 2015.

'Number of UK homes with TVs falls for first time', BBC News, 9 Dec 2014.

Timsit, Annabelle, 'Smartphones are disrupting the crucial connections between parents and their babies', qz.com, 31 July 2019.

Widdicks, Mary, 'Parental guilt is a cultural epidemic. It's time to let go of who we "should" be', *Washington Post*, 21 Aug 2019.

'How blue light affects your eyes and brain', Levin Eye Care, 12 Mar 2018.

'Night terrors and nightmares', NHS UK, 10 Aug 2018.

Bradshaw, Janssen, '7 tips for toddler quiet time', Everyday Reading.

Suni, Eric, 'How much sleep do we really need?', Sleep Foundation, 9 Mar 2021.

Dauvilliers, Yves and Tafti, Medhi, 'The genetic basis of sleep disorders', *Current Pharmaceutical Design*, 14(32), 2008, pp. 3385–95.

Caird, Ann, 'The barrier to calm bedtimes: the forbidden hour of sleep!', Attachment Parenting UK, 12 Dec 2017.

Suni, Eric, '12-month sleep regression', Sleep Foundation, 2 Oct 2020.

Wapner, Jessica, 'Are sleep regressions real?', *New York Times*, 15 Apr 2020.

'Chronic insomnia: why we lose sleep over it', BBC News, 14 May 2018.

'Sudden Unexpected Infant Death and Sudden Infant Death Syndrome', Centers for Disease Control and Prevention, 30 Sep 2020.

'It takes a village', Wikipedia.

'Elimination communication', Wikipedia.

Novak, Sara, 'Tips on starting potty training', What To Expect, 27 June 2018.

Bonebrake, Alan, 'Why do we sweat when in pain?', Quora.com, 2018.

'All About Allergies', KidsHealth, Oct 2016.

Gissler, Mika, Kaila, Minna, Lundqvist, Annamari, Metsälä, Johanna, Virta, Lauri J. and Virtanen, Suvi M., 'Mother's and offspring's use of antibiotics and infant allergy to cow's milk', *Epidemiology*, 24(2), 2013, pp. 303–9.

'How to spot those sneaky sources of gluten', Cleveland Clinic, 4 Mar 2020.

Tee, Anita, 'How I discovered – and solved my histamine intolerance for good', factvsfitness.com.

Lew Nolte, Dorothy, 'Children learn what they live – A Poem', Marigold Elementary School.

Bhurgava, Sumit, 'Diagnosis and management of common sleep problems in children', *Pediatrics in Review*, 32(3), 2011, pp. 91–9.

Dauvilliers, Yves, Maret, Stéphanie and Tafti, Mehdi, 'Genes for normal sleep and sleep disorders', *Annals of Medicine*, 38(8), 2005, pp. 580–9.

Honaker, Sarah, 'Should I wake my child up at the same time each morning?', Pediatric Sleep Council.

'Sleep matters: The impact of sleep on health and wellbeing', Mental Health Foundation, May 2011.

'How lack of sleep can affect gut health', Henry Ford Health System, 24 Feb 2021.

'New study points to another possible correlation between sleep and overall good health', Science Daily, 28 Oct 2019.

'Prevalence', Dr Schär Institute.

'The Allergy Explosion', Natasha Allergy Research Foundation.

'Definition: Histamine', KidsHealth.

Metsälä, Johanna, Lundqvist, Annamari, Virta, Lauri J., Kaila, Minna, Gissla, Mika and Virtanen, Suvi M., 'Mother's and offspring's use of antibiotics and infant allergy to cow's milk', *Epidemiology*, 24(2), 2013, pp. 303–9.

David Foulkes, *Children's Dreaming and the Development of Consciousness*, Harvard University Press, 1999, p. 52.

Alison Scott-Wright, *The Sensational Baby Sleep Plan*, Bantam Press, 2010, p. 1.

Xaviera Plas-plooij, Frans X. Plooij and Hetty Van De Rijt, *The Wonder Weeks*, Countryman Press, 2019, p. 21.

Marion Ingerson-Heart, *Sunshine 4 Your Soul*, Balboa Press, 2019, p. 30.

Christine Gross-Loh, *The Diaper-Free Baby*, William Morrow Paperbacks, 2007, p. 102.

Rebecca Chicot, *The Calm and Happy Toddler*, Vermilion, 2015.

Richard Ferber, *Solve Your Child's Sleep Problems*, Vermilion, 2013.

Joanna Faber and Julie King, *How to Talk So Little Kids Will Listen*, Piccadilly Press, 2017.

Acknowledgements

Wow – what a journey! Writing this second book without my late mum by my side (as she was for the first) has been quite a challenge. How amazing, though, to find my mother's words still ringing in my ears and hear her tutting at every grammatical mistake! Thanks, Mum, you've still been with me all the way through and I hope you will be proud of this book.

After struggling to believe I could do this alone, my love, thanks and gratitude go to those special people in my life who convinced me it was possible: to my daughter, Chelsea, who understood what an emotional journey this would be – you have been a constant source of support to me throughout and I'm deeply grateful. To my son, Jamie, who said with unwavering belief, 'You're going to smash it, Mum. Four months to write it? You only need two!' Your love and support are truly wonderful and more than appreciated. My sister Marion, who still tirelessly promotes my first book, supports me in so many ways and continuously endorses my work, telling all those who will listen – and even those that won't! My sister Jenny, who has expressed such a deep and heartfelt pride in all I have achieved and reminded me to keep the faith – in myself. To Becky, who is indispensable in helping to run The Magic Sleep Fairy, brilliantly manages my social media, expertly rescues all my technological crises and who compiled my sources – huge thanks!

Holing up with me in Turkey as I wrote this book, my love and thanks also go to my husband, Berkan, and to our great friend Necdat, for looking after me so beautifully. It's been a lonely journey at times, and being able to walk together on the beach each morning and evening has kept my spirits soaring. Special thanks, too, to Millie Mackintosh for writing such a lovely foreword and for the continuing endorsements of my work. My thanks also go to all the team at Transworld, Penguin and Random House who have worked under tricky circumstances and within a very short time-frame to bring this book to life. Special thanks to Alex Newby for the copy-editing and to Lizzy Goudsmit, my wonderful editor.

Immense thanks to all my wonderful clients and followers, many of whom have become very dear friends. Your continued endorsement, support of my work and purchase of multiple copies of my *Sensational Baby Sleep Plan* for all your pregnant friends (which pushed it to the number-one bestseller spot) has directly led to the commission of this sequel. I am truly humbled by the many messages of thanks, your brilliant stories of how my advice has helped and your unwavering trust in adopting, following and believing in my ethos, all of which inspires me to keep doing what I do. For the referrals, the recommendations, the poop pictures and more – I thank you all!

Index

acid-reflux *see* reflux
ADHD (attention deficit
    hyperactivity disorder) 19–21,
    225
adrenaline 113, 218
aggression 52, 130, 132, 221, 226
allergies 92, 129, 131, 228–51
    causes of 233–4
    diagnosing 234–5
    digestive discomfort 116–17
    foods causing 233–4
    gluten 231–2
    long-term solutions 241–2
    managing dietary changes 236–7
    sleep problems caused by 105
American Academy of Pediatrics 11
amygdala 28–9, 30
anaphylactic shock 228
antibiotics 127, 250
    and cow's-milk-protein
        intolerance 236
antihistamines 233

anxiety 13, 68, 112, 137
    and night-time waking 92
    separation anxiety 32, 92, 116–17
apps 56
attention 33, 109, 112
    attention span 220–1
    positive 10
audiobooks 58, 86, 140, 190, 191,
    248
autism 21

babies
    signs of good sleep in older
        babies 14
    signs of good sleep in younger
        babies 13–14
    signs of sleep deprivation in
        older babies 12
    signs of sleep deprivation in
        younger babies 12
    sleep cycles 17, 95
    sleep requirements 16

see also 6–12 months; 12–18
  months
bad breath 221
bathtime routines 10, 84, 88–9, 136–7
  siblings and 190
bed-wetting 206–7, 210
bedding 132
  potty-training 207
bedrooms
  curtains 19, 136
  preparing 136
  sharing with parents 73–4, 158–9,
    180–1, 182–4
  sharing with siblings 136, 153,
    192–3, 211
  temperature 19
beds
  making safe 131–2
  sleep-training toddlers in 159–64
  transitioning from a cot 91, 131,
    147–9, 152, 159, 182, 183–5, 211
bedtime 10, 18
  aggression at 132
  bringing forward 84, 198
  fears 70, 95–8, 120
  'forbidden sleep zone' and 87,
    88–9
  late bedtimes 9, 167
  Magic Sleep Fairy's bedtime
    rules 141–3, 147, 150, 177, 193,
    195
  managing with more than one
    child 189–91, 211
  natural bedtimes 167
  other people helping with 185–7,
    189, 211
  overstimulation and 113
  phobias of 74
  play before 88–9, 101, 137
  potty-training 207, 208–9
  promoting positive associations
    with 109–13
  refusals 153
  routines 73, 84, 88–9, 101, 113,
    136–7, 160, 207

rules 120, 141–3, 147, 150, 177, 193,
  195
screen time before 58, 88
  for toddlers with reflux 217,
    242–4
behaviour 130
  aggression 52, 130, 132, 221, 226
  behavioural development 30–2
  endorsing positive 48, 50
  explaining your 44
  focusing on 50
  issuing consequences for
    unacceptable 47–8
  repetitive or obsessive 224
  signs and symptoms of reflux
    217–28
biting 52
blackout blinds 136, 165
bloating 129–30, 229, 232
blue light 58, 139
books 35, 49, 108
  audiobooks 58, 86, 140, 190, 191,
    248
  libraries 53–4
bottle-feeding 219
boundaries
  accepting 45
  bedtime 72
  playdates 51
  setting 10, 23, 33, 34, 41–2, 44, 60,
    61
  transitioning to beds 159
bowel issues 221
brain development 10, 90
  cognitive development 26, 30, 36,
    39
  epigenetic adaptations 66
  reflux and 218
  REM sleep 17–18
breastfeeding 128, 188, 219
breast milk 127, 233
breath
  bad breath 221
  mouth-breathing 129, 218
bribes 107

calling out 218
calmness 10
Center on the Developing Child, Harvard University 65
challenging situations 130
    shielding children from 67
chicken pox 92
choking 223
chores 33, 35
chronic primary insomnia 68
circadian rhythms 16
climbing 42, 52, 224
clinginess 12, 116
clocks 86
    hour-change 105, 197–8, 211
    sleep-clocks 136, 139, 146, 147, 150, 153, 160, 164–5, 193, 197
clothes 224–5
co-sleeping 104, 107, 120, 160, 194
    on holiday 201
coeliac disease 229, 231
cognitive development 26, 30, 36, 39
colds 222
colic 116
comforters 98, 104, 118, 136, 138–9, 146, 150, 157, 165, 193, 221
conflict 45–7, 50, 89
congestion 222, 230
consequences, seeing through 47–8
consistency 44, 107–9, 125, 163
constipation 129, 221, 230, 232
contact-sleep 118, 119, 166
conversations 35–6
cortisol 8–9, 113
cot bumpers 157, 158, 159
cots
    sleep-training toddlers in 156–9
    transitioning to a bed 91, 131, 147–9, 152, 159, 182, 183–5, 211
coughs 222
    acid-reflux and 216
Covid-19 pandemic 80–1
cow's milk, transitioning to 93
cow's-milk protein allergy 194–5

cow's-milk-protein intolerance (CMPA) 127, 129, 213, 228, 229–31, 238–9
    and antibiotics 236
    congestion and 222
    symptoms 230
cravings 128
crying
    crying scale 76, 170–2
    crying to sleep 76–7
    during sleep-training 71, 72, 73, 151–2, 170–6
    overstimulation and 114
    reflux and 217
    separation anxiety 116
    sleep deprivation and 12, 13
    Toddler Tears and Tantrums scale 170, 172–3
    vomiting due to 174–5
cuddle-cushions 140, 146, 160, 165, 193
cuddly toys 98, 104, 118, 138–9, 153, 157, 160, 165
curtains 19, 136

dairy-free diets
    ingredients labels 237
    see also cow's-milk-protein intolerance; lactose intolerance
daytime naps 23, 82–5, 88, 153, 167
    benefits of 9
    inability to 218
    and night-time waking 91
    number required 78
    sleep-training for 165–6
    stopping 16, 80, 84–5, 198
daytime routines 18, 33, 113
    daily schedule 78–82
de-sensationalizing 137
delaying tactics 120, 161–2, 208
development 25–62
    behavioural 30–2
    developmental changes and sleep 63–7

developmental milestones 26–9,
   90–1, 217
genetics and environmental
   influences 64–7
diaries, food 250
diet 18
   changes to 92
   early waking and dietary
      intolerances 167
   effect of dietary issues on sleep
      116–17
   managing dietary changes 236–7
   offering healthy choices 45
   sleep deprivation and dietary
      issues 13
digestion 16, 128, 129
dirty hands 224
distal 215
DNA make-up 65–7
dopamine 56
dream feeds 104
dream pees 207–8
dreams, bad dreams, nightmares
   and night terrors 94, 95–9,
   116
drinking 128, 219–20
dummies 104, 119, 121, 138–9
   the 'dummy hunt' 145–6, 154
   reflux and 219
   removing 143–6, 147, 153, 154

ear-pulling 12, 129
early-morning waking 153, 166, 167
eating 219, 220
eczema 222, 230
18–24 months
   daily schedule 79–80
   daily sleep requirements 78
elimination-communication
   technique 201–2
emotions
   conflict 45–6
   emotional endorsements 10
   emotional milestones 26, 28, 29
   emotional regulation 28–9

endorphins 36
engaging with children 10
ENT (ear, nose and throat) issues
   223
environmental influences 64–7
epigenetics 65–7, 68
epigenome 65–6
exercise 10, 18, 115
expectations, setting clear 42
eye-rubbing 12

familial advanced sleep-phase
   syndrome 68
fatal familial insomnia 68
fathers, feelings of guilt 188
fears
   bedtime 95–8, 120
   night-time 69
feeding
   dream feeds 104
   feeding to sleep 118
   night-time 107, 118–19, 153, 155,
      167, 219
   sleep deprivation and 12, 13
fine motor skills 30
Five Cs 124, 125, 150, 151, 177
Five Ps 124, 125, 150, 168, 177
flushes 222
food, gagging or choking on 223
food allergies 92, 129, 131, 228–51
   causes of 233–4
   diagnosing 234–5
   digestive discomfort 116–17
   foods causing 233–4
   gluten 231–2
   long-term solutions 241–2
   managing dietary changes 236–7
   sleep problems caused by 105
food diaries 250
food intolerances 92, 129–30, 131,
   213–51
   causes of 233–4
   cow's-milk-protein intolerance
      (CMPA) 229–31, 238–9
   diagnosing 234–5

food diaries 250
gluten 231–2, 239–40, 242–3
growing out of them 238–40
lactose intolerance 228–9, 235
long-term solutions 241–2
managing dietary changes 236–7
poop and 221
reflux and 213–51
food-crams 223
'forbidden sleep zone' 87–9
formula 127
Foulkes, David 95
fresh air 10, 34, 114, 115
fruit 221
fun 34–5
furniture, climbing on 42, 52
fussy eaters 219, 245

gagging 223
games 36, 37–8
computer 56
gastro-oesophageal reflux (GOR)
213
effect on sleep 116–17
see also reflux
genetics 64–7
inherited sleep disorders 68
gluten intolerance and allergy
231–2, 239–40, 242–3
ingredients labels 240
symptoms 232
goddess mother myth 57
grandparents, staying overnight
with 185–6
gratification, regulating instant
56
grazers 245
greeting people 40
Groclock 139, 169
gross motor skills 30
growth and behavioural
development 11, 30–2
Guardian 2
guilt, parental 57–8, 67, 187–9
gut health 250

microbiome 235, 236, 241
and sleep 128, 129

habits
early waking 168, 169
encouraging good 41
hair-pulling 221
hands, dirty 224
happiness 10, 11, 34–5
head-banging 134, 154, 221
heartburn 116, 215, 216
histamine 233, 235
hoarse voices 222
holding, non-communicative 176
holidays 91, 105, 135, 182, 212
time-zones 198–201
Honaker, Dr Sarah 167
hormones
adrenaline 113, 218
cortisol 8–9, 113
dopamine 56
melatonin 8, 58, 88
sleep and 16
thyrotropin 88
tiredness and 12
hour-change 105, 197–8, 211
house, moving 91, 105
household rules 33–4, 41–2, 44, 60
hugs 10
hydrochloric acid 215, 222
hydrogen breath test 235
hyperactivity 130, 222–3, 225
ADHD and 20, 21

ignoring 225
illness 91, 92, 105, 131, 196, 223
immunity, sleep deprivation and
13
impulse regulation 29
independence 36, 45, 49, 61
insomnia 69
chronic primary insomnia 68
fatal familial insomnia 68
intolerances see food intolerances
irritability 12

kicking 52
Kids' Therapy Fund 188–9
Krishan, Dr Punam 81

lactase 228–9
lactose intolerance 228–9, 235
  symptoms 229
  testing for 235
language development 30, 35, 36,
  39
libraries 53–4
life events 56, 105
light sleepers 218, 225
lighting
  night-lights 98, 108, 139, 160
loudness 224
lower oesophageal sphincter (LOS)
  215, 216

Magic Dummy Fairy 144, 145–6
Magic Sleep Fairy's bedtime rules
  141–3, 147, 150, 177, 193, 195
manners 51, 60, 114
  encouraging good 38–41
  table manners 40
mealtimes 220
  table manners 40
  for toddlers with reflux 244–9
medication 240
melatonin 8, 88
  blue light and 58
mental health
  music and 36
  positive 39
  sleep and mental development
  11
Mental Health Foundation 77
milestones, developmental 26–9,
  90–1, 217
  0–12 months 26
  1–2 years 26
  2–3 years 27
milk
  breast milk 127, 233
  cow's milk 127–8, 31, 93

night-time feeds 104, 107, 118–19,
  153, 155, 167, 219
  when to stop milk feeds 80
misbehaviour 34
mistakes, learning from 61
monsters, fear of 96, 97–8
mood swings 13
morning wake-up management
  164–5
mouth-breathing 129, 218
mucosal membrane 216
music 36, 108, 114
  singing and signing 39

NAFA (Natasha Allergy Research
  Foundation) 233
nanny cams 86
nappies 202
naps see daytime naps
narcolepsy 68
National Library for Medicine 236
National Literacy Trust 39
nature versus nurture 65
newborn babies, sleep cycles 17
NHS
  ADHD report 20, 21
  sharing bedrooms with your
    baby 183–4
  transitioning to cow's milk 93
NHS Digital, sleep deprivation 2
night-lights 98, 108, 139, 160
night terrors 98–9, 116
night-time
  feeding 104, 107, 118–19, 153, 155,
    167, 219
  poops 205–6, 209, 210
  potty-training 205–10
  toilet regressions 210
  sweating at 218, 226
  waking 75, 91–5, 101, 153, 218
nightmares 95–8, 117
noise, white 19, 136, 139, 159, 160,
  165
non-coeliac gluten sensitivity
  (NCGS) 231

non-rapid eye movement (NREM) (quiet sleep) 17, 98
nursery, starting 91, 105, 135

obsessive behaviour 224
oesophagus 215–16, 220, 222, 241
older children
  signs of good sleep in 14
  signs of sleep deprivation 13
  sleep requirements 16
  see also 2–3.5 years; 3.5–5 years
omeprazole 194, 214, 226, 240, 241
one-to-one time 33, 55, 169, 181
overeating 219
overstimulation 113–15
  managing 114–15
  signs of 114
overtiredness 9, 18, 23, 104, 223
  epigenetic adaptations caused by 66

parents and parenting
  agreeing rules and strategies 41–2
  daily sleep requirements 77
  effect of anxiety and stress levels on sleep 68–70, 100
  parental circumstances 64–5
  parental guilt 57–8, 187–9
  'perfect' parenting 57, 67
  playdate strategies 51–2, 61
  positive and responsible 32–50, 60
  sleep deprivation 15, 100, 110–11, 124
  sleep disorders 68
Pediatric Sleep Council 166–7
'perfect' parenting 57, 67
perseverance 136
personality
  genetics and environmental influences 64, 65
  stubborn personalities 224
photographs 140, 142
physical contact 10

physical development 11, 26, 30
pickiness 224–5
play
  playdates 51
  pre-bedtime play 88–9, 101, 137
poop *see* stools
positive parenting 32–50, 60
potty-training 48–9, 211–12
  the basics 201–10
  night-time dryness 205–10
  night-time toilet regressions 210
  signs of readiness for 202–3
  toilet protests at bedtime 208–9
praise 48–9
  endorsing 60
  potty-training 204
prams, napping in 166
prefrontal cortex 29
premature babies 127
problem solving 33
promises, seeing through 47–8
proton pump inhibitors (PPIs) 240
punctuality 44–5

quality time 33, 36, 55, 181
quiet-time 16, 85–7

rapid eye movement (REM) (active sleep) 17–18, 95, 98, 116
rashes 222
raspy voices 222
reassurance sleep-training technique 123–78
  adapting to your needs 152–6
  basis of 124–5
  daytime naps 165–6
  early-morning waking 166
  health and safety guidelines 127–34
  morning wake-up management 164–5
  preparing for 126, 135–7
  setting the scene 138–49

tears, crying and tantrums
170–6
using the technique 149–64
reflux 74, 92, 128, 194–5
bedtime and sleep for toddlers
with 242–4
and cow's-milk-protein
intolerance (CMPA) 230
digestive discomfort 116–17
early waking and 167, 169
effect on sleep 116–17
fussy eaters and 128
mealtimes for toddlers with
244–9
medication 240
and night terrors 98–9
noisy breathers and 129
reflux explained 215–16
signs and symptoms of 128,
216–28, 244–5
sleep problems caused by
104–5
undiagnosed 131, 132, 133
see also food allergies; food
intolerances
repetitive behaviour 224
requests, being direct with 50
respect 60
encouraging 38–41
responsible parenting 32–50
rest, importance of 11
restless sleepers 219
reward charts 108
role models 44
routines 23
bathtime routines 10, 84, 88–9,
136–7, 190
bedtime 10, 18, 73, 84, 88–9, 101,
113, 136–7, 160, 207
daily 10, 18, 33, 78–82, 113
disruptions to 92
overstimulation and 114
potty-training 207
rules
household 33–4

Magic Sleep Fairy's bedtime
rules 141–3, 147, 150, 177, 193,
195
playdates 51
running 220

safety guidelines, implementing
43–4
school, starting 105
scratching 154, 221
screen time 10, 19, 54–9, 61, 92, 190
before bed 88–9
parental supervision,
authorization and control
58–9, 61
quiet-time and 86
second wind 87
self-esteem 60
boosting 181
self-harm 132, 154, 221
self-soothing 75, 117, 168
sense of belonging 33
separation anxiety 32, 92, 116–17
sharing 52–4
shared viewing experiences 55–6
shouting 224
siblings 64, 122, 180–96
arrival of 91, 105, 180–9, 210, 211
bathtime 190
managing bedtime with more
than one child 189–91, 211
parental guilt 187–9
sharing bedrooms 136, 153, 192–3,
211
sleep-training with more than
one child 136, 191–6
transitioning from cot to bed for
182, 183–5, 211
signing 39–40
sitting still 220
6–12 months
daily schedule 79–80
daily sleep requirements 78
daytime naps 82–3
skin, problems with 129, 222

sleep
daily schedule 79–82
daily sleep requirements 77–8
daily sleep requirements (6–12 months) 78
daily sleep requirements (12–18 months) 78
daily sleep requirements (18–24 months) 78
daily sleep requirements (2–3.5 years) 78
daily sleep requirements (3.5–5 years) 78
daily sleep requirements (parents) 77
developmental changes and 63–101
effect of parents' anxiety and stress on 68–70
epigenetics and 66
'forbidden sleep zone' 87–9
and gut health 241
healthy sleep habits 33
importance of 7–24
increase in childhood sleep problems 2
night-time waking 91–5, 101, 153, 218
parents' 17, 18, 77
promoting positive associations with 109–13
reflux and 217, 226
signs of good sleep 13
sleep cycles 8, 17–19, 98, 116
sleep hygiene 18–19, 23
sleep regression 90–1, 101, 116, 251
sleep requirements 15–16
sleep science 8–16
sleep-training 71–7
for toddlers with reflux 242–4
understanding common sleep issues 116–20
why sleep problems happen 104–15
see also daytime naps
sleep apnoea 99, 218
sleep-crutches 104, 117–20, 121, 128, 196
substituting 138–40
see also cuddle-cushions; dummies
sleep deprivation 2, 132, 166, 167
and ADHD 19–21
older babies and toddlers 9, 11–13
parents 15, 100, 110–11, 124
signs and symptoms of 11, 12–13
stress levels and 66
younger babies 12
sleep disorders, inherited 68
Sleep Foundation 15
ADHD and sleep deprivation 19
sleep-clocks 139, 146, 147, 150, 153, 160, 164–5
hour-changes 197
older children 193
sleep-training 71–7, 100
daytime naps 165–6
early-morning waking 166
importance of parental unity 135, 177
myths 73–7
night-time 123–65
preparing for 102–22
reassurance sleep-training technique 123–78
tears, crying and tantrums 170–6
with more than one child 191–6
'sleepy-time' message 149, 150, 151, 153, 158, 161, 177
smartphones 54, 55
smiling 34–5
snacks 19, 52, 219
snoring 129
social development 30–1
socialization 50–4, 114, 225
social media 56, 57, 236–7

solids 223
  introducing 128, 217
soya beans 230, 231, 234
speech development 35, 36, 39, 133
  delayed 222
stimulation, over- 113–15
stool acidity test 235
stools
  and cow's-milk-protein
    intolerance (CMPA) 230
  food intolerances and 221, 228–9,
    230, 232
  and gluten intolerance and
    allergy 232
  gut health and 128–9
  lactose intolerance and 228–9
  night-time 205–6, 209, 210
story-time 147, 160
stress 13, 57, 68, 112
  and night-time waking 92
  and toilet regression 210
stubbornness 224
sugary treats 19
sweating 218, 226

table manners 40
tablets 54, 55
talking to your child 38–9
tantrums 47, 221
  during sleep-training 170–6
  Toddler Tears and Tantrums
    scale 170, 172–3
technology 54–9, 61
  parental supervision,
    authorization and control
    58–9, 61
  technoference 57
teething 91, 93, 105, 196, 223
Tel Aviv University 20
television 54–5, 92, 114
  and bedtime fears 70, 88–9, 98
temperature
  bedrooms 19
  body temperature 98
three-strike rule 46–7

3.5–5 years
  daily schedule 79–80
  daily sleep requirements 78
throat infections 223
thyrotropin 88
tidying up, playdates 52
time management 44–5
time-zones 105, 198–201
timers 86
tiptoes, walking on 224
tiredness 12, 13, 219
  overtiredness 9, 18, 23, 66, 104,
    223
Toddler Tears and Tantrums scale
  170, 172–3
toddlers
  daily schedule and sleep
    requirements 16, 78–80
  development 25–62
  developmental milestones
    26–9
  growth and behavioural
    development 30–2
  naps 82, 84–5
  signs of good sleep in 14
  signs of sleep deprivation 11–13
  Toddler Tears and Tantrums
    scale 170, 172–3
toilet training 48–9, 201–10,
  211–12
tone of voice 35
trauma 91, 130
  childhood 69
  shielding children from 67
travelling 91, 105, 135, 212
  games 36, 37–8
  time-zones 198–201
  travel sickness 225
trust 47
12–18 months
  daily schedule 79–80
  daily sleep requirements 78
  daytime naps 82
twins 191–2
  development of 65

personality 64
sleep-training 154–6
2–3.5 years
daily schedule 79–80
daily sleep requirements 78
daytime naps 83, 84–5
two-way sound monitors 156,
162

under-mattress breathing sensors
158, 218
urinary tract infections 210

vaccinations 135, 229
video monitors 94, 147, 157
supervising via 86
vocabulary 39, 158, 161
vomiting 215, 223
due to crying 174–5
travel sickness 225

waking
dream pees 207–8
early-morning waking 153, 166,
167
morning wake-up management
164–5
natural wake-up time 167
night-time waking 91–5, 101, 153,
218
walking on tiptoes 224
water 128, 219–20
weaning 128, 217, 223
weight issues 220
white noise 19, 136, 139, 159, 160,
165
Who Knows Best: Can't Sleep Kids
154–6
wind 129–30, 229, 232
The Wonder Weeks 27
World Health Organization 157–8

About the Author

Alison Scott-Wright is a baby-, toddler- and child-sleep expert who also specializes in helping parents with the management of infant and toddler acid-reflux and associated dietary intolerances. For over twenty-five years she has worked 'hands-on' with families, sharing her knowledge and expertise with her clients and, most importantly, bringing sleep to thousands of homes. Fifteen years ago, one client named her the Magic Sleep Fairy and the name stuck – in fact, it became the trademarked name of her ever-expanding consultancy business, through which Alison continues to provide practical help, invaluable advice and much-needed support to parents around the world. She is a mother and a grandmother – known by her grandchildren as Mops – and she divides her time between her homes in Turkey and on the south coast of Dorset.